D1239801

9001002092

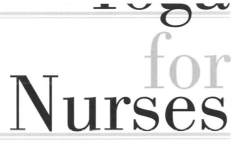

Yoga for Nurses

Ingrid Kollak, Dr. phil., RN, was educated and worked as a nurse in Germany, where a registration system is not common. She studied literature, sociology, and pedagogy at the Ruhr University in Bochum and spent time studying and researching in Paris (1984–1985), Vienna (1989–1990), and Providence, RI (1991–1993). In 1995, she became a professor in the health and nursing management programs at Alice Salomon University of Applied Sciences (ASFH) in Berlin. Since 2005, she has also been a licenced yoga teacher with the accreditation of the German and European professional boards of yoga teachers (BDY/EYU).

She has had two recent research grants. The first is for *Developing the Nursing Capacity for International Health Care Leadership,* Atlantis —Cooperation in Higher Education and Vocational Training (2007–2010), funded by the U.S. Department of Education's Fund for the Improvement of Postsecondary Education (FIPSE) and the European Commission's Directorate General for Education and Culture (DG EAC). The second is for *The Effects of Yoga on Patients with Mammacancer* (2008–2009) funded by the German Statutory Health Insurance (AOK).

For Springer Publishing Company she coedited with Dr. Hesook Suzie Kim two editions of *Nursing Theories—Conceptual and Philosophical Foundations.* Her recent publications are on *Burnout and Stress* (2008) and *Intercultural Perspectives in the Social and Health System* (2008). Since 2002, Dr. Kollak has been coeditor of *Pflege & Gesellschaft* (*Nursing & Society*), the theoretical journal of the *German Society of Nursing.* In January 2004, she began writing a monthly yoga column in the German journal *Heilberufe* (Healthprofessions).

She enjoys offering classes on theory, culture, and open yoga classes.

Yoga for Nurses

Ingrid Kollak, Dr. phil., RN

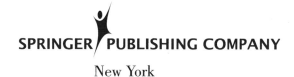

SPRINGER PUBLISHING COMPANY

New York

Springer Publishing Company, LLC
11 West 42nd Street
New York, NY 10036
www.springerpub.com

Acquisitions Editor: Allan Graubard
Project Manager: Barbara A. Chernow
Cover design: David Levy
Composition: Agnew's, Inc.

08 09 10 11/ 5 4 3 2 1
Ebook ISBN: 978-08261-38330

Library of Congress Cataloging-in-Publication Data

Kollak, Ingrid.
   Yoga for nurses / by Ingrid Kollak.
     p. ; cm.
   Includes bibliographical references and index.
   ISBN 978-0-8261-3832-3
   1. Yoga—Therapeutic use. 2. Nurses—Diseases—Exercise therapy. I. Title.
   [DNLM: 1. Yoga—Nurses' Instruction. 2. Self Care—Nurses' Instruction. QT 255
K815y 2009]
   RM727.Y64K65 2009
   613.7′046—dc22
                                                  2008037763

Printed in Canada by Transcontinental Printing.

To all friends of Doña Florina

Contents

Foreword by Jill Howie Esquivel, RN, PhD   ix
Acknowledgments   xi
Introduction   xiii

1   Common Health Problems of Health Professionals   3

2   How Yoga Works   7

3   A Short History of Yoga   13

4   Some Yoga Essentials   17

5   On Your Way with Yoga   23

6   Yoga Exercises at Work   29

7   Exercises at Home   79

8   Advanced Yoga Practice   147

9   Concentration and Meditation   187

10   Addresses and Literature   195

Index   197

Foreword

Yoga for Nurses presents nurses with a way to care for themselves as nurses and as persons. Although we are fortunate to live in an age of tremendous advances in health care and most of us can look forward to longer lives and better technology to make us more comfortable, nurses will continue to provide professional care as they have—pacing frantic hallways of hospital corridors and comforting families in intensive care units crowded with equipment and emotion. This care and the attention provided will continue throughout the night shift. Nurses, too, will work until later in life and carry the burden of their own illnesses as they care for their patients.

Each day, patients make intense mental, physical, and emotional demands on their nurses. Observing human suffering and mental anguish prods nurses toward patient advocacy, an effort that is continual and unending. The substantial physical requirements demanded of nurses are further compounded by the nurse-facilitated diplomacy orchestrated between care providers and families. Navigating the spiritual needs of patients provides yet additional opportunities for holistic caregiving.

Yoga, an ancient philosophy, is most often used in modern times to improve health and fitness. Yoga not only improves strength and flexibility, but it provides a venue for meditation and relaxation. More researchers are beginning to investigate the effects of yoga and have demonstrated how yoga alleviates health problems, such as hypertension and chronic back pain. *Yoga for Nurses* offers a practical "how-to" that addresses both the mental and physical parts of our bodies. In this book, you will find yoga exercises that can either be integrated into your workday or done at home. Advanced yoga practice techniques are presented for those who desire more challenges.

As health professionals, we need to support ourselves as we face the challenges found within our chaotic work environments. Providing care to ourselves during off-work times can seem elusive, but caring for ourselves in the health care environment can be virtually impossible.

Yoga for Nurses provides the means by which nurses can support and enhance their ability to care for themselves. It gives nurses information and strategies they can use to deal with the physical and mental imperatives found in their daily work life. Just as a new parent embraces a guide for baby care, nurses will welcome a way to care for and improve their physical and mental health.

Jill Howie Esquivel, RN, PhD
Nurse Scientist
Associate Clinical Professor
University of California, San Francisco

Acknowledgments

This book has grown out of my practice, teaching, and research of yoga in diverse settings: in yoga schools, clinics, and universities, as well as conferences and retreats.

I could not have written this book without the help of friends and scholars on both sides of the Atlantic. Special thanks go to Allan Graubard, my acquisitions editor, who believed in this book. His publishing expertise, as well as his knowledge and experience as a yoga practitioner, helped me to write an easy-to-read book with proven exercises.

I am grateful to my yoga teacher Edel Hausch, as well as to Liliana Velasquez and Bouba Kaba, who modeled for most of the photographs in this book. Additional thanks go to Jeanne Ayoko Abbey, Astrid Deingruber, Konrad Liesenborghs, Astrée Oberlaender, and Charlotte Pöhlmann – colleagues from the Westend Clinic, who became yoga models for the photographs on the title and chapter pages. I also want to thank the photographers: Donald Becker (photos of all exercises), and Ali Ghandtschi (full-size photos).

I want to thank Shannon Pfohman for help with some of the translations. Special thanks go to Arnd Kilian who read all the drafts, polished my words and sentences, and helped to make this an enjoyable book to read.

Introduction

Nature has provided us with remarkable bodies fit to adapt to many challenges. While modern life takes care of many of our immediate needs, it still exposes us to environments in which we experience physical and mental stress. This is particularly true when working in demanding fields such as health care.

Mental pain and chronic pain are among the highest ranked reasons for failures and breakdowns in the workplace. The high technical and communication demands, the necessary team work and individual responsibilities, the need to talk to other professionals as well as to patients and their families and friends, the long hours of walking along corridors or standing in operation theaters, the heavy lifting of patients, and the motionless sessions in front of a computer screen occupy us throughout the work day. Health professionals often suffer chronic pain in the neck, sometimes accompanied by headaches and sore eyes, or their lower backs hurt and their legs feel heavy and hard to move. Work stress leading to an inability to consciously alternate between states of high energy and profound relaxation disturbs the sleep–wake rhythm and leads to being wide awake at night and feeling groggy in the morning.

As health professionals, we all need ways or techniques to support us and enhance our ability to physically and mentally rise to the challenges of our jobs. Short breaks for yoga exercises (asana) can fit into the work routine and provide quick help. Indeed, yoga is able to both prevent and cure the symptoms and illnesses that are the result of pain, whether mental or physical. Yoga works physically to reduce pain by stretching and strengthening muscles made tense from our normal work routines, which have their strenuous and repetitive movements. Additionally, yoga also works on a mental level by providing an exceptional anti-stress program. Yoga exercises combine movements and breathing rhythms that not only make the workout easier but also calm the mind and help us to focus.

In this book, you will find yoga exercises that either can be included in your work routine or done at home. All yoga postures are detailed with their corresponding breathing techniques. They are explained step by step in the text and are illustrated by photographs. This way, you can exercise on your own and in diverse settings. If you begin yoga and would like to practice in a group, there are the many yoga classes and teachers available in your locale from which to choose.

- **Yoga at Work:** Yoga exercises during small breaks in work can increase your energy, vitalize your mind, relax your body, and help your concentration. To help you find suitable "yoga postures," the postures are presented within an anatomical and physical framework. Together with synchronized breathing and enhanced by regular practice these asana produce a positive and immediate effect and can be done almost anywhere.

- **Yoga at Home:** To deepen the effects of the short yoga routines, comprehensive exercises with lasting effects that are easier done at home than in a work environment are presented. This way you can systematically exercise from head to toe. You learn diverse postures and breathing exercises (pranayama) while doing yoga at home and deepen your knowledge of how to energize your body and relax in different ways.

- **Advanced Yoga Practice:** As an ambitious yoga practitioner, you may want to try out some challenging asana and learn more about their effects. This book provides information on special yoga asana and how they work. They are organized along the yogic classification of forward, backward, and sideward bends, upright and inverted postures, and twists and balancing postures.

- **Concentration and Meditation:** To complete your exercises, this book provides information on how you can develop your own practice of concentration and meditation and let it become a part of your individual yoga program. In relaxing and balancing asana, you learn to visualize and listen to better focus your attention.

This book is a practical "how-to" guide to using yoga to manage stress and relieve pain while gaining the strength necessary to work best and longest with patients and colleagues. It provides knowledge about the effects of yoga, helps each person find the right style, and teaches you how to start an individual yoga program at work as well as away from work.

Yoga
for
Nurses

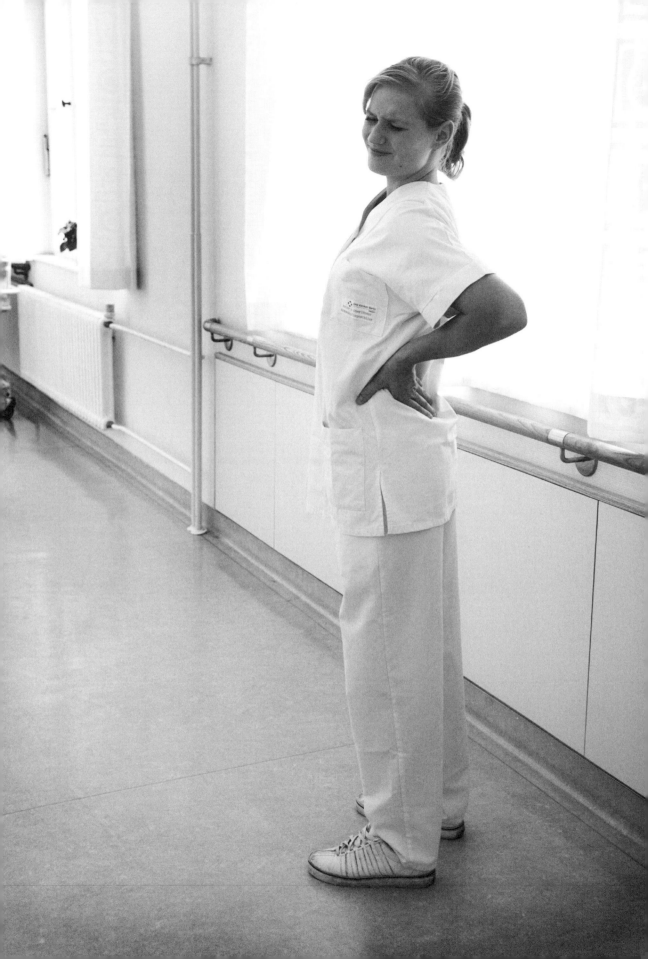

Common Health Problems of Health Professionals

1

Muscle pain and stress are two common problems encountered by health care professionals as a result of increasing work loads and constant challenges. Stress and muscle pain are two problems that often go hand in hand. Even though these problems are widely spread and experienced by many workers in the health care setting, people afflicted with them often feel misunderstood, especially if their problems are lasting. The attitude of co-workers may also change. People with long-term afflictions suddenly seem to be less stress resistant and less robust. The problem is not their weakness in regard to stress, but their inability to regularly relax and repeatedly gain strength.

The feeling of being stressed has two consequences. The first is constantly tightened muscles. For example, tight shoulder muscles can lead to a stiff neck, which can result in headaches. You may become reluctant to move your head and shoulders, but resting them in the incorrect position only worsens the condition. The second is a propensity to brood, which can lead you to misinterpret questions about your condition and feelings. You may find yourself skewing your communication with colleagues or clients. When communication with those you work with and work for becomes a burden, you feel more and more isolated, and your stress will increase.

You may know a lot of people who often talk about stress, and you may have lost all perspective about what is good for you and when things are becoming too much. While there are numerous definitions of stress, most of them conclude that stress is a result but not a cause. The good news is that you can fight stress by changing your attitude, but you have to find the specific reasons that have caused you to feel stressed. Since people in the same setting are affected differently by the same challenges, there might be better ways for you to handle the situation. Some people seem better at avoiding stress or interpreting situations differently; they seem to know and use proper techniques. Another important fact is the support or pressure of the work environment. The settings vary widely for health care professionals. You might be a member of a highly specialized team in clinic settings or be completely on your own in home care settings. You might be running your own business and fear that you cannot afford to take time off. Or you might be working in alternating work shifts that makes it difficult to obtain proper rest.

Stress is a normal hormonal reaction that leads to increased pulse and breathing rates, to tight muscles, and to focused attention. This mobilization of your physical and mental resources prepares you to act in challenging situations. It is helpful if the requests are on the same level as the resources. Unfortunately, they are not always in proper balance. This is why symptoms of stress are common to everyone. Most people have experienced situations in which they overreacted or felt overburdened. Some people become sick if these experiences are lasting or if they do not know how to react differently or to change the situation. Feelings of being overloaded with work or lacking time for yourself can lead to aggressive thoughts or behavior, as well as feelings of anxiety and panic.

In our field, heavy or improper lifting and carrying and long hours of standing and walking often generate back pain. Constant muscle pain can lead to poor posture and reduced movement in an effort to avoid the pain. But these may exacerbate the underlying cause. Expecting any movement to be painful causes you to avoid all movement; as a result, your whole body becomes stiff and sore. In trying to meet your obligations, you do not take enough time and do not ask for assistance.

Short vacations or sick leave will not help in the long run. Drugs and medicines help only in the beginning, but only become another burden if you become used to them or addicted to them. You have to find a proper level of self-care that both reduces your vulnerability and enhances your resilience. The diverse yoga postures presented in this book will help you to better relax your body and mind and be stronger physically and mentally. Yoga exercises dissolve joint blockages and help you become more flexible and stronger. They break the vicious circle of stress and help you to calm your mind and become focused.

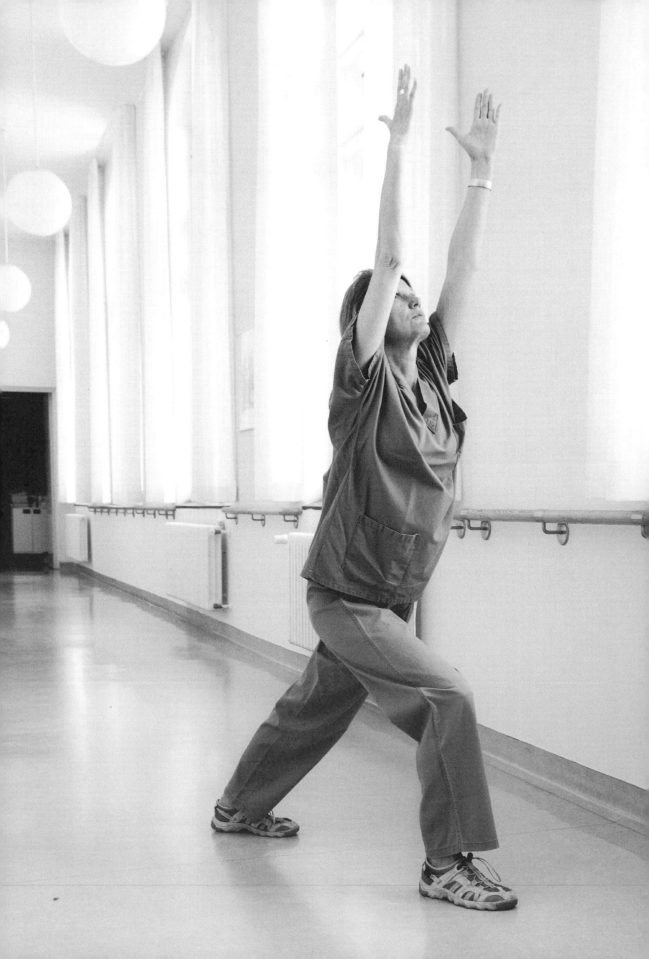

How Yoga Works

2

Yoga has an effect on the body, mind, and soul. It addresses both somatic as well as emotional afflictions that can arise from stress and poor posture. Backaches, tight muscles, and tension headaches can be remedied by yoga exercises. Yoga also helps alleviate recurring troubling thoughts that create fear, sadness, or aggression. When practicing yoga, the connection between the physical body and the spiritual condition becomes obvious.

Yoga can become an antidote to either inactivity or overactivity. For example, if you practice dynamic yoga, you can relieve the stress that comes from sitting or listening for long periods of time. If you practice relaxing yoga, you can compensate for overexertion. The effects of each exercise—which will be discussed subsequently—can be felt immediately. If these yoga exercises are practiced regularly, they can also replicate lasting antistress treatments and result in greater flexibility and strength. Yoga positively benefits everyone.

Yoga and the Musculoskeletal System

It is obvious that yoga postures, asana, require muscular effort. The muscle activity can be measured on different levels. A high degree of muscle activity increases the energy exerted, resulting in greater oxygen intake as well a higher pulse rate and more frequent breathing. Muscles that do not exert strength on immediate activity possess tension in the form of an elastic countermovement or tension in posture. Measurements of pulse rate, breathing frequency, and muscle tension for most of the well-known postures show that yoga belongs to the type of workout with less impact. Yoga has a great influence on the body, but with less stress on the body. Furthermore, comparisons between experienced and inexperienced yoga students show that an economization of muscle activity enters into play. The level of effort will be reduced as soon as you are able to achieve a certain posture, thus enabling more concentration when carrying out an exercise (cf. Ebert, 2003, pp. 275–285).

As your knowledge and experience grow, you will find that your enjoyment of yoga increases. Your concentration will be enhanced, but with less stress on your muscles. The same thing is true for your breathing, which becomes more even and regular. On the other hand, it is obvious how focused and physically fit competent yoga students are. You will find that regular repetition of the postures will become more stimulating. This is because you learn more about your body and your well-being when practicing the exercises, thus resulting in more enjoyment.

Yoga and Body Awareness

Receptors in the muscles, joints, and skin provide information about joint positions and associated muscle activities, as well as about strength and stretching conditions, pressure and tension, influences of temperature, and characteristics of the skin surface. These receptors send stimulants to the brain, which then registers and identifies the source. Through the practice of yoga you learn a lot about your own posture. As a result, bends and twists of the body stimulate the sensory cells of the organ of equilibrium in horizontal or vertical directions. The comprehensive movements of your body and the changing positions of your head when practicing yoga train you to become more conscious of your own spatial orientation. Learning to be cognizant of body temperature, of strain and relaxation, as well as of stretching and bending, increases your sense of body awareness. In this way, you learn to notice poor posture when you are not practicing yoga and you can make adjustments whenever necessary.

When practicing yoga on a regular basis, you exercise all joints and learn to avoid poor posture. By intentionally relaxing those muscles that you are not using, you learn to more frequently attain a relaxed posture in yoga as well as in your everyday life. The better you synchronize your breathing and moving, the more profound your musculoskeletal relaxation will be in phases of breathing exhalation. Tension and relaxation are constantly alternating. With the conscious coordination of breathing and movement, yoga helps you to counteract lasting tension. If you feel your shoulders are tense and pulled up you can relieve the tension by exhaling. The brain registers the varying stimulators, identifies their locations, and trains your body in awareness: a challenging stretch, a flowing movement, a relaxation that comes with an exhalation, the composition of different body surfaces, as well as fine temperature differences. Practicing yoga results in an effect similar to receiving a good massage.

Yoga and the Inner Self-Attention

If you constantly run at "high speed," you will not be able to push yourself any further or are likely to pay for your permanent stress overload with poor health. Creating a balance between tension and relaxation and between exertion and recuperation is an art form that can be learned through the practice of yoga. While practicing yoga, you become more and more aware of your body and your physical well-being. You learn to detect poor positions and to respond to stressful situations. You navigate through different kinds of obstacles and learn more about your resources. An improvement in body awareness enhances your ability to understand yourself. Focusing your attention on your own body will allow you to sense your powers. This can be manifested as increasing attention to your own thoughts during yoga practice, as an awareness of your musculature during certain exercises, and as a mood that you feel when ending a position. The main thing is the degree to which you can focus your awareness. Yoga exercises offer the chance to do things differently, to leave behind your usual thoughts, and to experience a sense of joy instead. "Yoga is bhoga" (joy) is a well-known saying. It means that whoever perceives the effects of yoga on the different levels of feeling and understanding enjoys its physical and mental pleasures. These effects transpire during the exercises and extend beyond the time of exercising.

Yoga and Self-Efficacy

Subjective certainty is understood as self-efficacy, as being able to master basic requirements and to reduce stressful situations. It can first be observed when learning and practicing yoga exercises regardless of the level of ability of a person to master such situations. A playful approach in dealing with these requirements is good practice for everyday situations. Yoga will be more rewarding if you practice it with less stress and with less exertion. The more you focus on your breathing and moving, as well as on proper alignment, the more you learn how to rely on yourself. The certainty of being able to rely on your own abilities and resources grows along with the experience needed to successfully master all kinds of challenges.

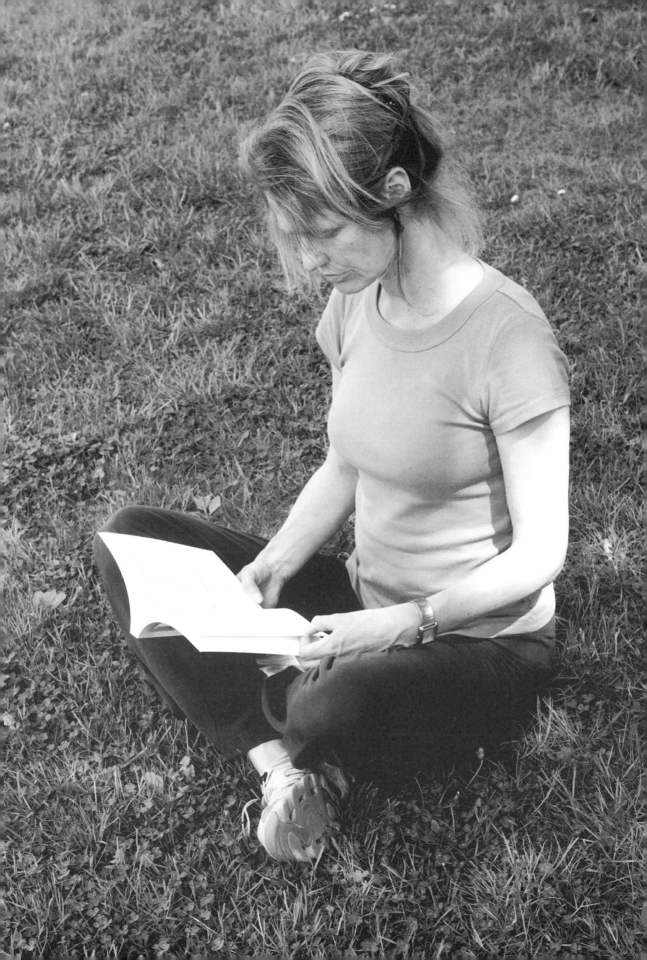

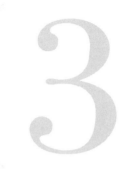

A Short
History
of Yoga

"Yoga practice offers the foundation to understand and develop yoga. Whoever practices yoga attentively can practice it for a long time and enjoy it." This is a liberal translation of a central passage from the yoga sutras, an approximately 2000-year-old Sanskrit text from which a first systematic yoga depiction has remained unchanged. Yoga tradition is even older and uses a large number of postures, called asana, to bring body, thoughts, and feelings into accord over and over again. Asana release blockages in the joints and ease and invigorate the musculature, foster attentiveness and open and deepen breathing spaces, and enable room for new thoughts and the ability to concentrate on the essential.

Yoga helps and discloses itself only through its practice. Therefore, you should start directly by doing the exercises; you will find that the changes in your own body will provide you with a lasting impression of its effectiveness. Motivated by your own experience, the theoretical foundation of yoga can thus be understood. The wealth of literature on yoga is expansive, offering a wide variety of directions to deepen your knowledge. The following section contains an initial introduction to yoga.

Today most people think of yoga as acrobatic positions. Headstands or the lotus posture could even be synonyms for yoga. This style of yoga, which attempts to achieve a consciousness of your own body, however, is relatively new. In the beginning, the center of yoga was based on spiritual-religious being. It was all about the transition of the body and complete spirituality, which were achieved by concentrating on meditation and prayer. Yoga is closely associated with Brahmanism, a religion previously connected with Hinduism. Postures became a central theme only because of their connection with an ability to maintain a meditative or prayer position motionlessly and for a long time. Documents on yoga from this era extend back to the Rig-Veda of the Keshin-Hymnus, approximately 1200 years before, and the Yoga Upanishad, 1600 years after, the beginning of our calendar time.

To a certain degree the prominent trend in yoga today, Hatha Yoga, more likely represents the opposite of the previous approach. Rather than focusing on overcoming the body, in Hatha Yoga the body and its well-being are at the center. This approach, in which yoga is considered physically uplifting, can be understood when taking into account the influence of old folklore traditions, which also have an influence on Indian religions. But while much is known about yoga through texts written by priests, historical sources of Hatha Yoga are sparse. However, the orientation toward the body was combined with the philosophic and religious roots of yoga and thus created a visual language describing the body as a "temple of God" or as "a place of pilgrimage and blessedness." Besides the Patanjali Yoga Sutras, written roughly 2000 years ago, the main texts of Hatha Yoga are the Yoga Upanishads (written 500 years after the beginning of our calendar time), the Goraksha-Shataka (written 1200 years after the beginning of our calendar time), and the Hatha-Yoga-Pradipika (written in the fifteenth century).

The historical developments of yoga can be traced back to well-known Sanskrit texts as well as to today's Indo-European succession languages, leading to the following division:

- Archaic or Proto-Yoga (3000–1800 years before our calendar time) mentioned in the Vedic collections
- Preclassical Yoga (approximately 1500 years before our calendar time) documented in the early Upanishads
- Epic Yoga (500 years before our calendar time until 200 years after our calendar time) known from the Mahabharata—one of the two central Indian folklore epics (besides Ramayana) along with the well-known Bhagavad-Gita—as well as from the Upanishads of that time
- Classical Yoga (at the beginning of our calendar time) in Patanjali's Yoga Sutras
- Postclassical Yoga (approx. 200 to 1900) depicted in the Yoga Upanishads, Goraksha-Shataka, and the Hatha-Yoga-Pradipika
- Modern Yoga with various schools and ensuing literature

Georg Feuerstein, who suggested this division in his *Encyclopedia of Yoga*, ends his explication with the following sentence: "Other classification systems are possible" (2000, p. 125). Indeed, Feuerstein uses the term "classical" in regard to Hatha-Yoga. Linguists might use the term "classical" when referring to Sanskrit texts on yoga some thousand years ago.

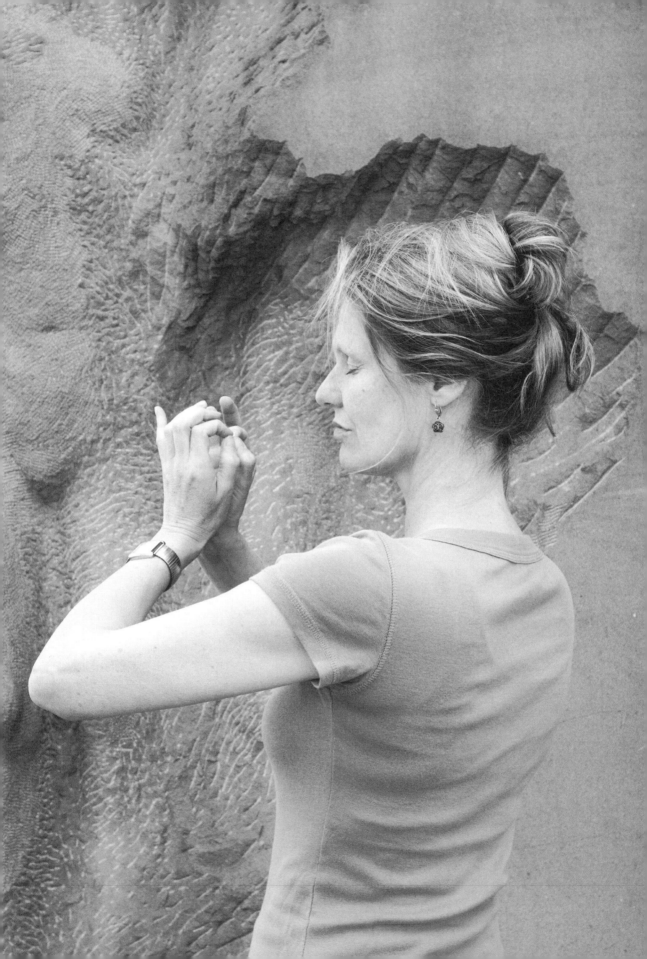

Some
Yoga
Essentials

4

Yoga Is for Everyone

Yoga practice can be quite diverse: You will find it in senior citizen homes and kindergartens, with dancers and office clerks, as Power Yoga or as a support for cancer therapy. It simply depends on which form of yoga fits a particular person. Since yoga courses are now offered everywhere—in city adult education centers, in schools and companies, in sports clubs and spas, and last but not least in yoga schools—it is easy for you to attend a yoga class and then come to your own decision.

Since yoga is currently "in," there are many class options and advertisements. They convey an image of the different styles and forms of yoga as well as the different traditions associated with these styles. The web pages of the best known Hatha Yoga traditions are listed at the end of this book. Learning the way yoga teachers live and convey this tradition can be observed only through personal experience.

You will also find that it is easy to do "Yoga in between" at work. Develop your yoga practice for small breaks. Learn a set of asana and try it out at work. This way you can do yoga at any time and any place, independent of groups and teachers.

Retain a Flowing Motion

Yoga postures have become part of sports and gymnastics classes, including the candle, the quadruped stand, and the bridge. They have also been integrated into new types of workouts, such as Pilates training. Compared to yoga, however, a clear difference can be seen in the breathing technique. When practicing yoga, breathing should be even, complete, and synchronous with the movement. If you increasingly lower your shoulders with every exhalation, you will not only feel the stretching in the shoulder musculature, but will also relax, placing your weight on the ground, i.e., maintain no unnecessary muscle tension and feel relieved as a result. This feeling can activate and spread new energy. You can also activate this feeling at any time by combining exhalation closely with the intention to relax your shoulders: A person practiced in yoga notices if the shoulders are pulled up and tensed and is able to loosen and relax the shoulders with an exhalation.

Breathe In and Out Through Your Nose

To maintain a fluidness of breathing and movement over long stretches of practicing yoga, it is essential to evenly breathe in and out through the nose. This breathing provides the necessary strength to get into the posture, to stretch the muscles, and to hold the positions. The breathing also shows the amount of energy necessary for a posture. You should never be out of breath while practicing yoga. Always practice on a level that allows you to evenly breathe. There are breathing exercises that make the fluidity of breath audible and clarify whether breathing and movement are proceeding synchronously. Some yoga schools use humming sounds to let you sense the synchronicity of breathing and moving. The sound should be audible to the very end of the movement. You can try the effect and hum "hmm" and if you like it make it part of your yoga practice. Conscious breathing also helps you to stay focused. Notice how long you can focus on your breath streaming past your nostrils. Do not think about the time you are unfocused; rather keep noticing the time when you were highly concentrated.

There are also breathing exercises in quiet positions that foster vitality, increase blood circulation, and improve oxygen supply, or that influence the pressure in your belly and help you digest. During these breathing exercises you sometimes inhale through your nose and exhale through your mouth. There are only a few exercises in this book using these techniques. The breathing prevalent in yoga and in this book, though, is a noiseless, even, and complete breathing in and out through the nose.

Develop Your Own Yoga Practice

Practicing yoga regularly is the key to success. It is ideal to regularly practice at the same place and at the same time. In this way, improvements, current strengths, and weaknesses become evident.

If you practice yoga directly after waking up, you build yourself up for the whole day: stretch your muscles and tendons, move your joints, increase your blood circulation, and become aware of your well-being, your thoughts, and your feelings.

A regular visit to a yoga class during the day is also a treat. This is ideal for either interrupting or ending your working day as yoga mobilizes strength needed to carry out additional tasks either in a professional manner or for leisure activities.

At work you can carry out exercises on your own. Standing or seating postures are well suited for short interruptions of your daily work routines. When done intermittently during the working day yoga exercises can lower stress levels, improve physical well-being, and increase concentration levels.

Slow and relaxing yoga exercises are suitable for the evening or before going to bed. They help you to tune down and to find peace and quiet.

Whatever agenda you decide on, you should keep to a fixed time for your yoga practice and not constantly change the schedule. If you repeatedly wonder whether now or later is a good time or if there is enough time or if more time might be needed, or if your desire to exercise is strong enough or might eventually increase later on, you will waste time in unproductive thinking and create even more stress for yourself. It helps if you just do your yoga at a fixed time and recognize what it does for you. You will always feel better once you got going. Enjoy yourself with the help of yoga.

Cultivating Your Yoga Style

Developing a conscious individual yoga practice is vital. Yoga starts with practicing and understanding the postures and counterpostures. At the beginning, keep to a fixed rhythm: Always start the exercises from the same side of the body. In the Hatha-Yoga-Pradipika all exercises begin on the left side. Repeat the exercises at a constant length. Start with six complete inhalations and exhalations, which equal six complete movements.

If you are able to do the postures you will experience the changes in the dynamic and static forms of the postures. Yoga can fuel your blood circulation and raise your blood pressure if you use dynamic forms and yoga can lower your blood pressure if you use a relaxed form. If you do not suffer from specific illnesses, a combination of alternating exercises that challenge you with new and difficult postures and relax you with easier and well-known postures is a good mixture. A change between learning new postures and repeating the well-known ones might be similar to the tasks you encounter in everyday life. This further enables you to better deal with unusual situations or routines.

Continuously practicing yoga postures and deepening your understanding of their significance allow you to adapt postures to your needs. Experienced yoga students know when they need a special stretch, an extra bend, or a certain resting posture. To become an expert it is vital that you practice yoga with consciousness. Right from the beginning keep to your yoga time and to your rhythm and learn to listen to your body.

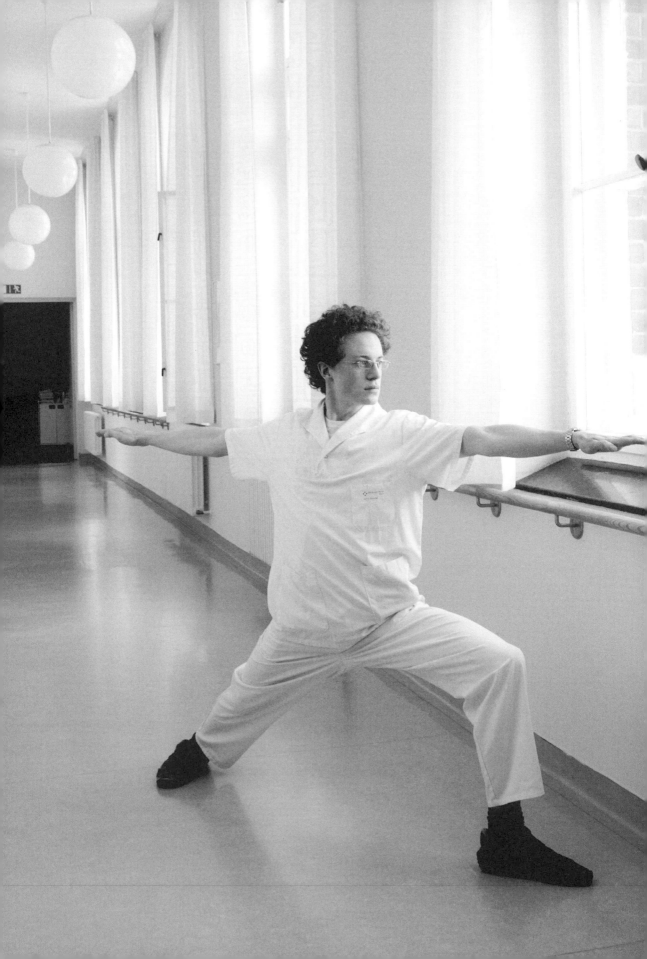

On
Your Way
with Yoga

5

Practical Tips

Easy accessibility of your place for yoga is important because practicing regularly is paramount, whether at work, at home, or in class. If at work, using a yoga mat may not be feasible, but the exercises described in Chapter 6 of this book certainly are. At home, of course, place your mat within reach so it is ready to use. You can also look for a yoga class near where you work or live. Keep a copy of the description of your actual yoga postures at work to sustain continuity among work, home, and class.

Good teachers are important because they are supposed to motivate and lead you. Anyone who feels stressed and has a sore back should be reaffirmed, supported, and feel relief of their pain through yoga. Teachers should convey confidence and positive self-esteem and should help you to dissolve joint blockages and to steadily build up muscles and become more flexible and stronger. There are minimum standards for the education and qualification of yoga teaching. The professional organization of yoga teachers has a list of trained yoga instructors should you want one. Yoga group size and individual support are important factors as well, since yoga is expected to adequately convey how to handle your body, your thoughts, and your feelings in order to be able to fend off stress and prevent muscle pain. This coincides both with good instructors and a protective setting. "Appropriate responses to a class should be invigoration, calm, and satisfaction. Inappropriate responses would be stress, agitation, or physical discomfort" (Carrico, 1997, p. 39).

Comfortable clothes are important as well. Sports clothes such as pants and t-shirts are okay as the clothing should feel good and sit well. Yoga is practiced with bare feet. This way you can feel your weight evenly distributed on your soles, strengthen your feet muscles, feel the outer sides of your feet on the ground while you are shifting the weight, and so on. Another important reason is that it reduces the danger of slipping. At work you can practice yoga in your normal working clothes and shoes as long as they feel comfortable and allow some stretches and bends. If it is appropriate you can take off your shoes. Be careful not to slip.

While a nonslip yoga mat is fine as it is warm to the touch and provides support, even a blanket can be used at the beginning for the relaxing breathing exercises and then rolled up as a knee cushion. Certain yoga traditions and schools use a lot of props. You do not need to buy them. Use them during the class, but at home you can replace them with books, belts, blankets, and towels. The fewer things you need, the easier it will be for you to begin. The aim is to be able to practice yoga everywhere. Do not worry too much about preparing and focus your energy on practicing yoga.

The Options of a Personal Journal

If you decide to learn and practice yoga, you might like to find ways to help you incorporate yoga into your daily life. A personal journal can be of help. Using this, you can document your plan of action as well as the progress you are experiencing. Your personal journal helps you to better understand your goals and options for achieving them, as well as the reasons for successes and failures. Therefore, your personal journal should have two columns. In one, note what you want to achieve and during what time. In the other column, write what you were doing, your thoughts, ideas, and comments. Your journal can be a booklet or a file on your computer.

You can write down the goals you want to achieve and the posture or a group of postures you want to learn, the time you want to practice, and the results you are looking for. While writing your individual action plan, think of the following:

- What do you want to achieve?
- Which asana are you going to practice?
- How often and how much do you want to practice?
- At what time do you want to practice?

Goals	Results

Ease the pain in the lower back.
Knee to the chest posture.
Twelve movements per session, two times per day during 1 week:
    After wake-up.
    Variation on the chair during morning break.
	Here you note how often you have practiced, the effects on your lower back, the enhancement of your flexibility, and the thoughts that you have when you are practicing.
	    Become aware of your progress and of obstacles in your daily practice.
	    Example: Missed my wake-up exercise because I stayed in bed too long. Since Thursday changed to bedtime exercises. Much easier to do! Back feels better after practicing at work and when lying in bed. Slept well!

You can also write down your goal and try out different ways to realize it.

Goals	Results

Ease the pain in the lower back.
Knee to the chest posture on a mat.
Twelve movements per session, two times per day during week 1:
    After wake-up.
    Variation on the chair during morning break.
	Write down your daily routine, the outcomes, and your thoughts and comments.
	    Example: The knee to chest posture helps a lot to stretch and get started. No back pain on Saturday after a 2-hour visit at the museum!
	    After some comments, Alex is exercising with me during morning break. Lots of fun. Maybe we will visit a yoga class in Alex's neighborhood.

Ease the pain in the lower back.
Folded leaf posture in bed.
Maintain the posture for 12 inhalations and exhalations per session, two times per day during week 2:
    After wake-up.
    Before falling asleep.
	Write down your daily routine, the outcomes, and your ideas and comments.
	    Compare the two yoga asana: the accessibility, the comfort, the warmth as a plus, the results, etc.
	    Example: The folded leaf posture is comfortable, but not as effective as the knee to the chest posture.
	    I am continuing the knee to the chest practice at work because of Alex.
	    At nighttime the folded leaf posture is a treat. I will continue with it as well as the knee to the chest in the morning. Have to think of a new yoga trick for Alex (eagle posture!).

A journal can help you to apply yoga to your daily life. It will help you to note a new competence, to stay on track regarding the outcome of your efforts, and to learn to use yoga as a way to enhance your well-being. If you can lower your stress level or reduce your back pain, you will gain energy and confidence. Do not expect too much but do not fail to note your progress and honor it.

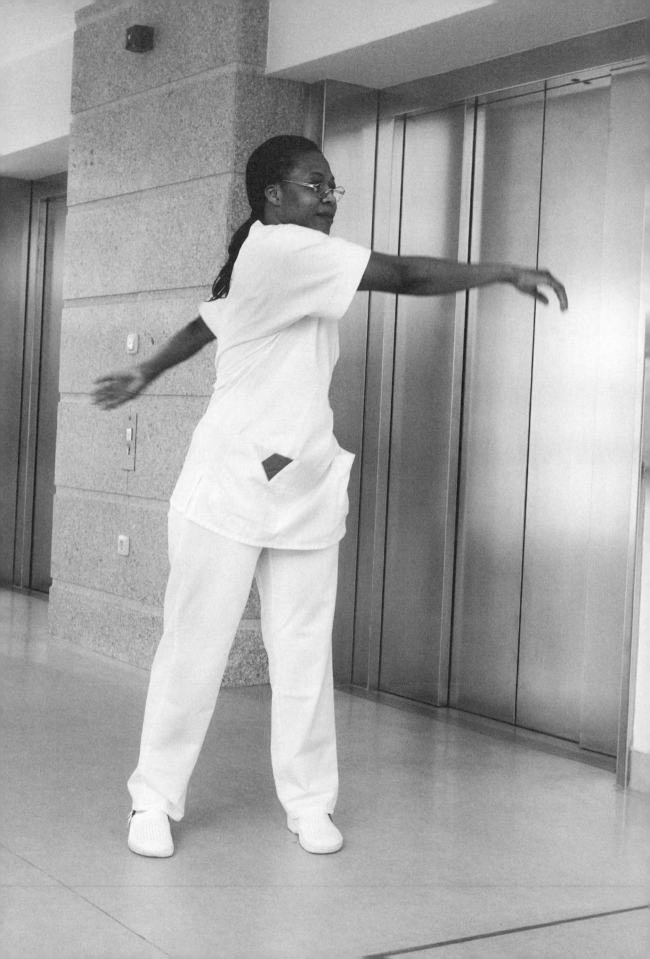

Yoga Exercises at Work

6

From Head to Toes with Consciousness

Use yoga exercises during small breaks at work. "Yoga in between" can help you to become balanced after a hard or single-sided workout, to bring up your energy and revitalize your mind, or to relax your body and concentrate. Develop your yoga practice: your special set of asana, your time and place, your rhythm, and your way of doing them.

To help you find the suitable yoga asana, the asana are anatomically organized from head to toes. Each asana focuses on the part of the body mentioned. Luckily, most of the asana also affect the body and mind in more than just one way, that is, eye exercises also help to calm the mind and shoulder exercises in a stand-up position also affect the legs, feet, and toes. Together with synchronized breathing and backed up by regular practice, these asana have a positive and immediate effect.

Note

The following exercises at work are suitable for beginners of yoga. Exercises having an effect naturally also possess a contraindication. The greatest problem is that beginners often overdo them. They want to learn yoga quickly and often think that they already know the asana. What they might know are modified versions of them. To do the asana in an effective way without harming yourself, you need to be aware of proper alignment as well as of proper breathing. The best thing to do is to focus your awareness on the effects of each asana. What does the asana do to your body and your mind? Does it feel good?

Special Considerations

- Pregnant women should do special yoga exercises and not simply use the exercises provided here.
- People with glaucoma, a detached retina, ear inflammation, or uncontrolled high blood pressure should keep their heads above heart level.

- If you feel acute pain, do relaxing postures and do not fight the pain.
- After surgery, restart your yoga practice slowly.
- If you have an abdominal hernia, any injury or inflammation in your back or abdomen, or if you have sciatica, consult your health care practitioner before you start practicing.

Yoga is for everyone. It is just a matter of finding the right postures and the right style for your individual condition. Become more and more aware of your body and mind and your physical and mental well-being while you are practicing. Learn to detect poor positions and to align your joints. Learn to identify high stress levels and to consciously alternate between tension and relaxation. Synchronize your breathing and moving. With the conscious coordination of breathing and movement, yoga helps you to counteract lasting tension and to reduce high levels of stress. Yoga is a rich and elaborate approach to health and well-being—and yoga is joy (bhoga).

Remember

Inhale and exhale through your nose during the yoga exercises. There are only a few exceptions (see Chapter 7: "Yoga Exercises at Home") and these are clearly marked. To develop your own rhythm of practicing yoga, always start the exercises from the same side of the body and repeat the exercises for a constant length of time.

All Postures at a Glance

Indications	Goals	Name of Posture
Get Started	Two Basic Stances for All Exercises	Standing Posture, Seated Posture on a Chair
Headaches, Stiff Shoulder and Neck	Relieve Tension	Elephant Posture, Head Rotation, Head Bow, Easy Turtle Posture
		(continued)

Indications	Goals	Name of Posture
Burning Eyes	Keep Your Eyes Moist	The Lying Eight, Near and Distant View, Cupping and Blinking
Poor Posture of Shoulders and Upper Back, Hurting Wrists	Stretch and Relax	Arm Rotation, Great Gesture, Torso Rotation, Hand Gesture, Hand Lotus
Lower Back Pain	Build Muscle Strength	Easy Mountain Posture, Forward Bending Posture, Triangle in Motion
Stiff Knees, Tired Legs and Feet	Rotate, Bend, and Lift	Knee Rotation, Runner Posture, Palm Tree Posture
Little Energy and Poor Posture	Recharge and Increase Your Strength	Hero 1 Posture, Stargazer Posture
Moody and Feeling Blue	Lift Your Spirit	Bend and Twist, Hero 2 Posture
Low Concentration	Improve Memory and Stay Focused	Tree Posture, Alternate Nostril Breathing

Get Started: Two Basic Stances for All Exercises

The following basic stances are starting postures for all the exercises and poses that you can do at work. They help you to concentrate on your body and mind and to breathe properly.

These stances can also serve as relaxing postures before and after you are doing your in-between workout.

Last, but not least, these postures give you the time to feel the effects of an exercise. This might be after you have completed the whole session or an asana or the first half of an asana. In this case, you take up the basic stances. After you have practiced on one side and compare the feeling in both sides of your body before you continue and do the other side.

Standing Posture

- Position your feet hip joint width apart from one another. The outer edges of your feet are parallel to one another. The inner and outer edges of your feet are touching the ground, and the weight of your body is evenly distributed on your soles (Figure 6.1).
- Extend your knees (do not hyperextend them). Your thighs are rotated outward.
- Your pelvis is erect and your spinal column is stretched. Your sit bones point in a downward direction, while the crown of your head points in an upward direction.
- Your belly is relaxed. Your bottom, or rather your pelvis muscles, are tightened.
- Your sternum is raised and your shoulders and arms hang down loosely.
- Your chin is parallel to the ground, and your face, lips, and tongue are relaxed (Figure 6.2).
- Completely breathe in and out through your nose.

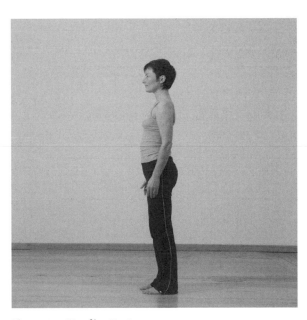

Figure 6.1. Standing Posture

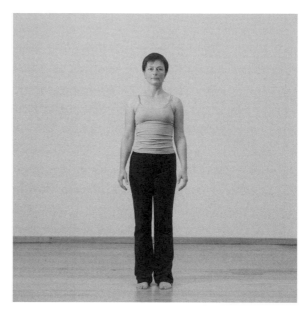

Figure 6.2. Standing Posture

Seated Posture on a Chair

- Take a seat and distribute your weight evenly on both sit bones.
- Position your feet hip joint width apart from one another. The outer edges of your feet are parallel to one another. Your knee joints are above your ankles.
- Your pelvis is upright, the entire length of your spinal column is stretched, and your head crown extends upward.
- Your sternum is raised, and your hands lay loosely on your thighs.
- Your chin is parallel to the ground, and your face, lips, and tongue are relaxed (Figure 6.3).
- Completely breathe in and out through your nose.

Headaches, Stiff Shoulder, and Neck: Relieve Tension

Often you are not aware that you are keeping your shoulders tight and in a pulled-up position for a long time. After a while you feel the tension, your shoulders hurt, and you develop a headache.

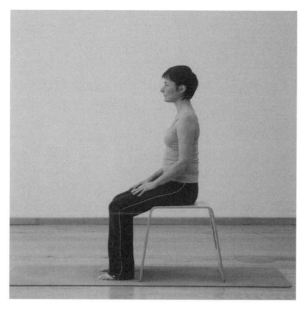

Figure 6.3. Seated Posture on a Chair

To prevent headaches that stem from tense shoulders and neck, relieve the tension with the following exercises. You can do the turtle posture to fuel the circulation of your upper body and get energized.

Elephant Posture

- Come into the standing posture (see "basic stances").
- Place your feet a little further apart (Figure 6.4).
- Inhale and swing your whole body to the left, lifting your right heel (Figure 6.5).
- Exhale and swing your whole body to the right, lifting your left heel (Figure 6.6).
- Imagine your arms are sleeves while swinging them from one side to the other. Steadily extend the movement to a maximum.
- Maintain the energy level for six full breaths.
- Gently slow down the movement until you stand in the initial pose.
- Bring your feet closer together and get back into the standing posture.
- Feel the effect of the movement. You may close your eyes if it is pleasant for you.

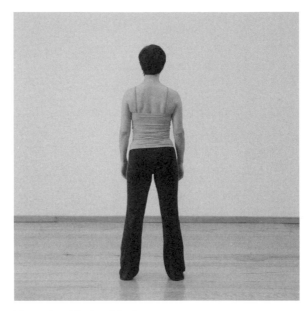

Figure 6.4. Elephant Posture

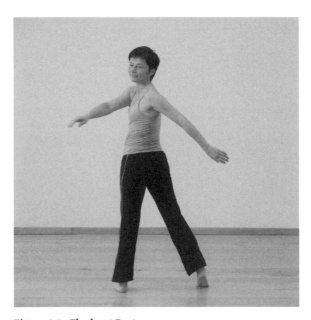

Figure 6.5. Elephant Posture

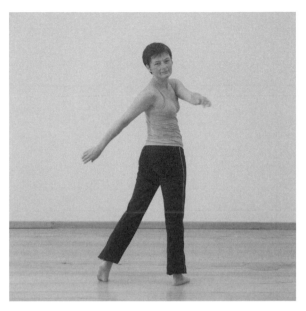

Figure 6.6. Elephant Posture

Head Rotation

- Come either into the standing posture or into the seated posture on a chair (see "basic stances").
- With an inhalation, turn your head to the right. Make sure that your chin is parallel to the floor, that your head does not bow, and that your shoulders stay relaxed (Figure 6.7).
- With an exhalation, turn your head to the left without bowing (Figure 6.8).
- Repeat the rotation for six complete inhalations and exhalations.
- Rotate your head into the middle and get into your initial posture. Feel the effect of the rotations. You may close your eyes if you like.

Head Bow

- Come either into the standing posture or into the seated posture on a chair (see "basic stances").
- With an inhalation, stretch your spinal column, stretch your neck, and keep your head in a stretched out position.
- While exhaling, gently bow your head to the right side. Your ear is getting closer to your shoulder. Make sure that both your shoulders stay relaxed (Figure 6.9).

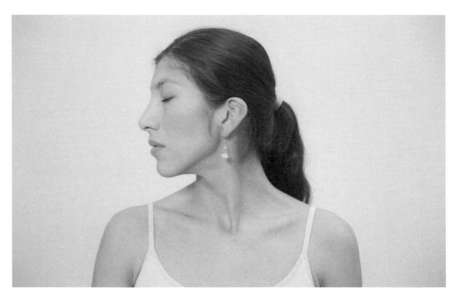

Figure 6.7. Head Rotation

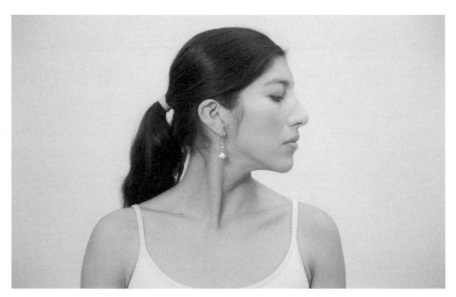

Figure 6.8. Head Rotation

- With an inhalation, slowly raise your head into the starting position.
- Exhale and gently bow your head to the left side (Figure 6.10).
- Slowly raise your head into the starting position with an inhalation.

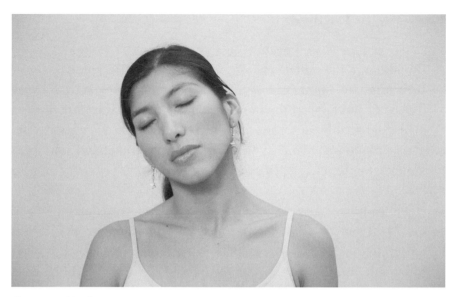

Figure 6.9. Head Bow

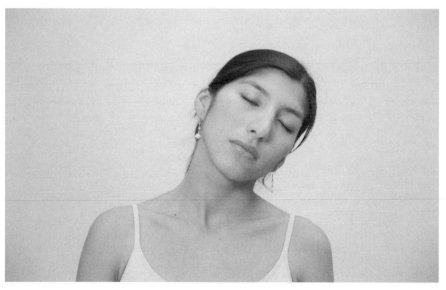

Figure 6.10. Head Bow

- Repeat the movements for six complete inhalations and exhalations on each side.
- Finally, get back into the seated posture and feel the effect of the stretches. You may close your eyes if you like.

Easy Turtle Posture

- Come into the seated posture on a chair. (see "basic stances").
- Breathing in through your nose, first, lengthen your spine.
- Breathing out through your nose, bend your upper body forward from your hip joints. (You may stop half way with your forearms on your thighs and rest for an inhalation.) Slowly, let your hands and arms sink between your knees toward the floor and bend your arms around your lower legs, placing your hands either next to or on your feet.
- Relax your head and drop your shoulders. Breathe completely and evenly in and out through your nose and hold this position for six complete inhalations and exhalations, closing your eyes if it is comfortable to do so (Figure 6.11).
- If you feel like responding after several breath cycles to an even greater stretch, then drop your upper body even more and reach for your toes with your hands.
- To release the position, inhale and raise your torso until you can place your elbows on your knees. Slowly roll up your body and return to the seated posture.
- Feel the effects of the inversion for a moment and, if it is comfortable for you, close your eyes.

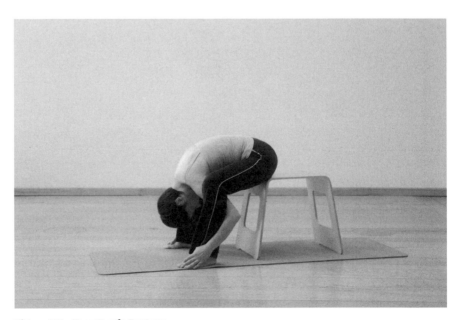

Figure 6.11. Easy Turtle Posture

Burning Eyes: Keep Your Eyes Moist

After hours of work in artificial light or after staring at a computer screen, your eyes feel itchy and burn and your vision becomes blurry. One reason is that you often do not blink enough; the other is that you do not alternate between near and distant viewing.

This is what you can do for your eye health during a short break.

The Lying Eight ✓

- Come into the seated posture on a chair or on the floor. (see "basic stances").
- Extend one arm to eye level, make a fist, and keep your thumb up.
- Focus on your thumbnail with both eyes. Hold your head in a fixed position and do not move it. Only the eyes move during this exercise, as they focus on and follow the movements of your thumb.
- Breathe out through your nose while lowering your stretched out arm, directing it downward (Figure 6.12) and along the lower right half of your peripheral view. Continue moving it completely to the right to a point at which your thumbnail is still visible (Figure 6.13). While breathing in through your nose, move your stretched arm up-

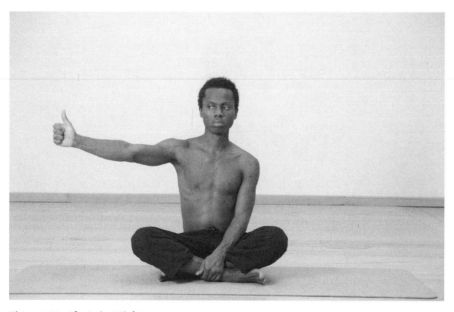

Figure 6.12. The Lying Eight

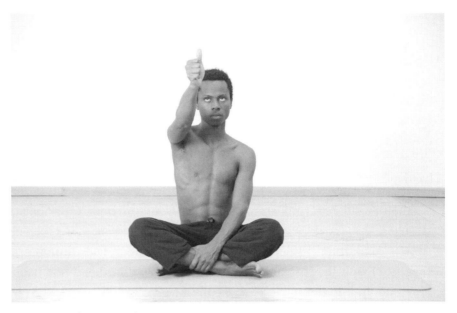

Figure 6.13. The Lying Eight

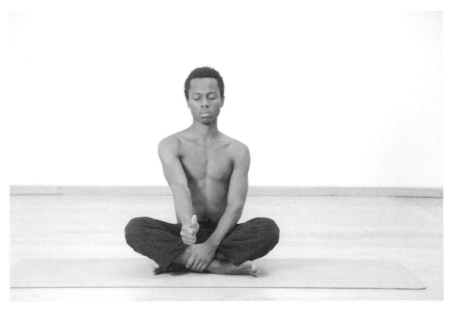

Figure 6.14. The Lying Eight

ward along the upper right half of your peripheral view (Figure 6.14) and proceed until moving back to the starting position.

- Lower your arm, bring your other arm up, and do the same exercise to the other side.
- Repeat the exercise three times on each side.
- Continue with the exercise "cupping and blinking" (see below).

Near and Distant View

- Come into the seated posture on a chair or on the floor (see "basic stances").
- Extend one arm to eye level, make a fist, and put up your thumb.
- Look at the tip of your nose and take a breath in and out.
- Look at your thumbnail and breathe in and out (Figure 6.15).
- Look at an object that is close by and breathe in and out.
- Look at an object in the distance and breathe.
- Next, with an inhalation, no longer lock your eyes on an object. Just look into the sky or ahead of you. Then breathe out again.
- Repeat each step in reverse order until you are looking at your nose again.

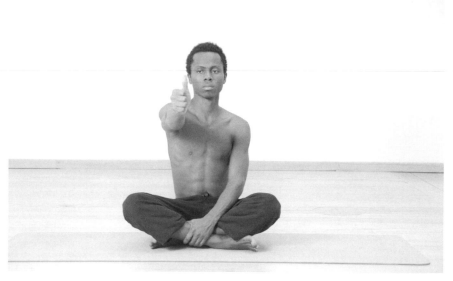

Figure 6.15. Near and Distant View

- Do the complete exercise six times.
- Continue with the exercise "cupping and blinking" (see below).

Variation: This exercise can be done discretely during the day—at work or even on the way to work while on the bus, train, or subway. In this case, focus on an object near you instead of on your thumbnail.

Cupping and Blinking

To help your eyes to stay moisturized and to really relax, the warmth from the palms of your hands can be transferred to your eyes and eye sockets.

- While your eyes are closed, rub your hands forcefully together until you sense the warmth (Figure 6.16).
- Completely cover your closed eyes with your palms—the fingers are upright against your front. Without any contact between your palms and your eyelids, feel the warmth being transferred and completely relax your eyes (Figure 6.17).
- After a while take your palms off, relax your arms in your lap, and keep your eyes closed.

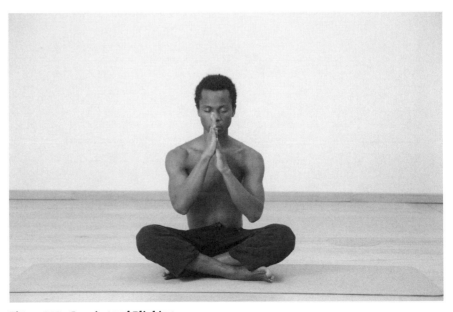

Figure 6.16. Cupping and Blinking

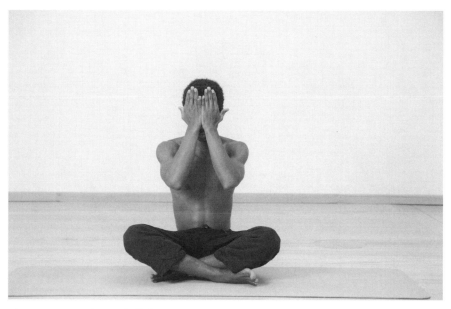

Figure 6.17. Cupping and Blinking

- Start blinking with your eyelids; change from quick blinks to slower blinks.
- Keep your eyes open at last, relax your whole body, and feel the effects.

Variation: When doing the eye exercises at home, you can do them in a seated position on your mat. With a forward bent you get a good stretch and you are able to rest your head.

- After rubbing and warming the palms of your hands, straighten your complete spinal column and breathe in. Breathe out and bend forward keeping the stretched out position, and set your elbows down on your mat. Your head rests against your hands while your eyes are covered by your warmed palms (Figure 6.18).
- Breathe in and come back into the starting position keeping your spine stretched out. Relax your arms and hands in your lap.
- Start blinking with your eyelids, changing from quick blinks to slower blinks.
- Keep your eyes open at last, relax your whole body, and feel the effects.

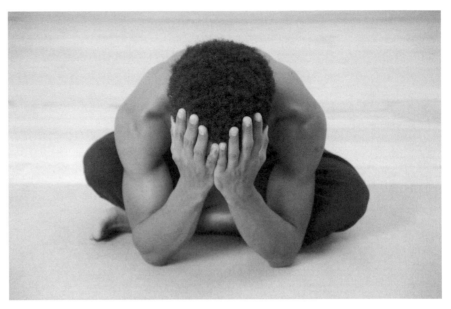

Figure 6.18. Cupping and Blinking

Poor Posture of Shoulders and Upper Back, Hurting Wrists: Stretch and Relax

Since our arms and hands work together most of the time, we tend to bend our shoulders forward. With this movement, we often tighten the chest, round our upper back, move our head and chin forward, and slightly nod backward. (Visualize a vulture to get the matching impression.) This hurts the upper spine in many ways and reduces breathing. It is necessary to regularly counter this by stretching and pulling the shoulders backward and sitting upright.

After long hours of typing or after heavy lifting and carrying, your wrists hurt and your fingers get stiff. Your wrists need some bends and your hands need some rest. Here is what you can do.

Arm Rotation

- Come into the standing posture (see "basic stances").
- While breathing in through your nose, slowly raise your arms sideways to shoulder height. Only raise your arms; make sure that you

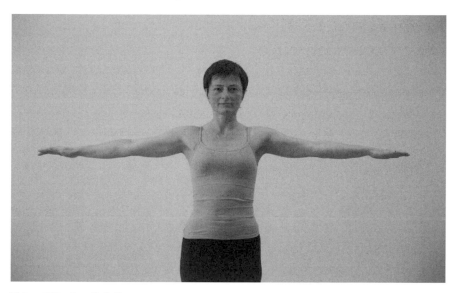

Figure 6.19. Arm Rotation

do not pull up your shoulders. If you are not exactly sure, pull up your shoulders briefly and let them sink again (Figure 6.19).

● With an exhalation, rotate your stretched arm backward until your palms are facing backward (Figure 6.20).

● With an inhalation, rotate your stretched arm forward until your palms are facing forward (Figure 6.21).

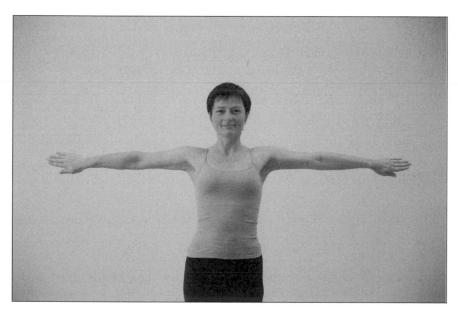

Figure 6.20. Arm Rotation

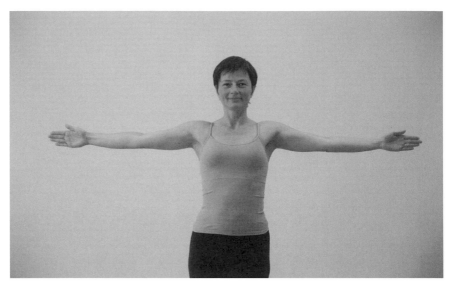

Figure 6.21. Arm Rotation

- Repeat this rotation of your stretched arms six times.
- With an exhalation, slowly lower your arms.
- In the standing posture, feel the effects. Close your eyes if it is pleasant for you.

Great Gesture

- Come into the standing posture (see "basic stances").
- Stretch out your arms and move them backward. Bring your hands together behind your back and cross your fingers—the palms are facing your back.
- Inhale through your nose and slowly raise your arms (Figure 6.22).
- Exhale through your nose and slowly lower your arms.
- Repeat the movements during four inhalations and exhalations.
- Maintain the posture during two inhalations and exhalations.
- With an exhalation, slowly lower your arms and return to the standing posture.
- Feel the effects of the back stretch—with your eyes closed if you like.

Variation: If you have strong back muscles and a flexible spine, bend your upper body further backward. Hold this backward bend for six full inhalations and exhalations.

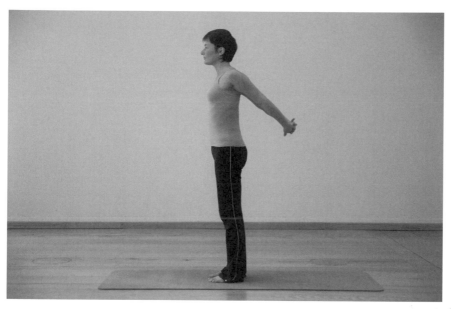

Figure 6.22. Great Gesture

Torso Rotation

- Come into the standing posture (see "basic stances").
- Breathe in through your nose and, parallel with your breathing, slowly raise both your arms over your sides to shoulder height. Only raise your arms; do not pull up your shoulders. If you are not exactly sure, you can pull up your shoulders briefly and let them sink again. Bend your left arm until your hand is in front of your sternum (Figure 6.23).
- With an exhalation, turn your stretched out right arm backward and rotate your upper torso and your head to the right, leading with your outstretched right arm (Figure 6.24).
- With an inhalation, rotate back into the starting pose and change the position of your arms: bend the right arm and stretch out the left arm.
- Breathing out, turn your head and upper body to the left, leading with your outstretched left arm.
- With an inhalation, turn back again, change the positions of your arms, and do the other side.
- Repeat this torso rotation six times.
- Finally, while in the standing posture, feel the effects of the rotation in your thoracic vertebrae. Close your eyes if it is pleasant for you.

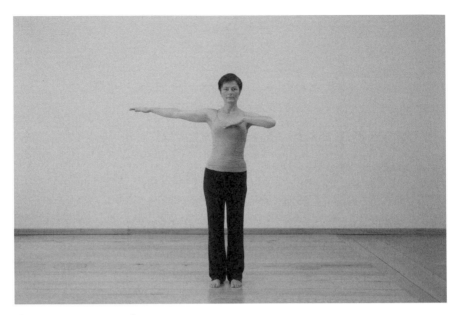

Figure 6.23. Torso Rotation

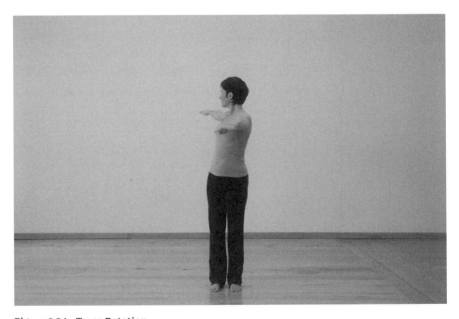

Figure 6.24. Torso Rotation

Hand Gesture

- Come into either the standing posture or the seated posture on a chair (see "basic stances").
- Inhale and lift your arms in front of you to chest height.
- Exhale while slowly moving your hands downward until your fingers are pointing to the floor (Figure 6.25).
- Inhale while slowly moving your hands upward until your fingers are pointing to the ceiling (Figure 6.26).
- Repeat the gentle movements for six full inhalations and exhalations.
- With an exhalation, lower your arms into your lap or to your sides and feel the effects of the upward and downward bends.

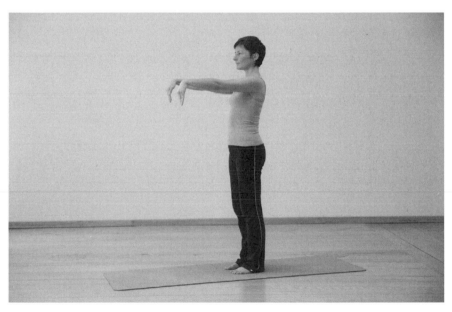

Figure 6.25. Hand Gesture

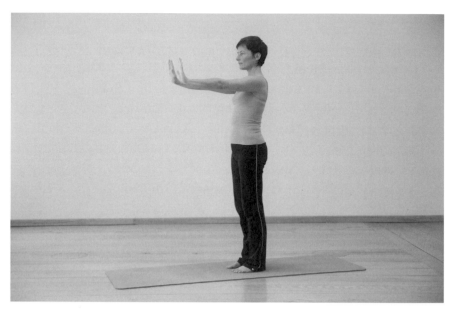

Figure 6.26. Hand Gesture

Hand Lotus

- Come into the seated posture on a chair. (see "basic stances").
- Lift your arms and elbows to chest height.
- Put the tips of both your index fingers and thumbs together to form a nice circle, and relax the other fingers.
- Bring the backs of both your hands together (Figure 6.27).
- Gently rotate your hands with forearms inward. Both wrists are moving gently around one another with the fingers alternately pointing downward and upward.
- Maintain the gentle move for six inhalations and exhalations.
- Then change the direction and gently rotate outward for another six inhalations and exhalations.
- You can do the exercise with your eyes closed.
- Lower your arms into your lap and feel the effects in your wrists.

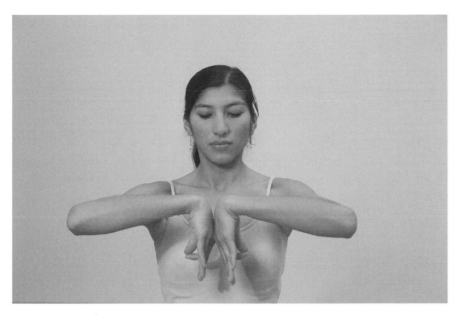

Figure 6.27. Hand Lotus

Lower Back Pain: Build Muscle Strength

Lifting and transporting patients strain back muscles and put heavy weight on the joints—especially if you suffer from exhausted trunk muscles, weak abdominal muscles, and have a poor posture. A good core stability, proper alignment, and muscle strength help to manage the load and to prevent joint inflammation and muscle spasms.

It is also necessary to practice yoga regularly at home to build up muscle strength. Exercises on the floor help to determine the proper alignment. A blanket provides warmth. The following exercises help you to keep your lower spine and pelvis aligned. They also give you a proper stretch forward. Since stretches to the side are rare in everyday life, it is necessary to regularly do them and keep the outer hip muscles flexible and in good shape.

Easy Mountain Posture

- Come into the standing posture (see "basic stances").

- Place a chair in front of you. Make sure the chair cannot slide away. Put your hands on the seat, stretch out your spine, and bend your knees.
- Exhale while slowly walking backward until your arms are fully stretched out and your hip joints, knees, and ankles are aligned (Figure 6.28).
- Stay in the position for six complete inhalations and exhalations.
- While inhaling slowly walk closer to the chair, bend your knees, and roll up into the standing posture.
- Feel the stretch of your arms, back, and legs. Close your eyes if it is comfortable for you.

Variation: If you suffer from glaucoma, a detached retina, ear inflammation, or uncontrolled high blood pressure, keep your head above heart level. Use the back of a chair as a prop (Figure 6.29).

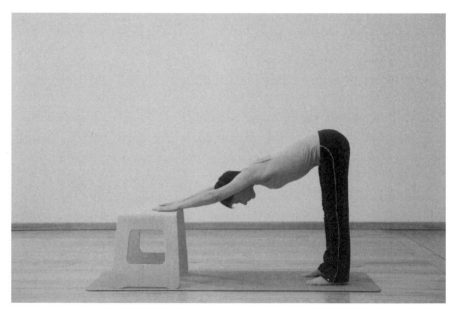

Figure 6.28. Easy Mountain Posture

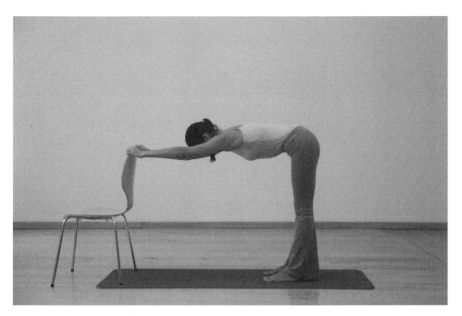

Figure 6.29. Easy Mountain Posture

Forward Bending Posture

- Come into the standing posture (see "basic stances").
- Put one foot forward. Make sure that your feet are still hip joint width apart and that the outer sides of your feet are parallel. Keep both legs stretched and both heels on the floor (Figure 6.30).
- With an inhalation, stretch your spine again.
- Exhale and slowly lower your torso, keeping both shoulders in a line (do not bring one forward) until you can put your hands on your front thigh (Figure 6.31).
- Maintain the position for six full inhalations and exhalations.
- With an inhalation, return to the starting position.
- Move your front foot backward and get into the standing posture.
- Close your eyes and compare both sides—both legs, both sides of your pelvis, and both sides of your face.
- Repeat the exercise on the other side.
- Finally, get into the standing posture, close your eyes, and feel the balancing effect of the whole exercise.

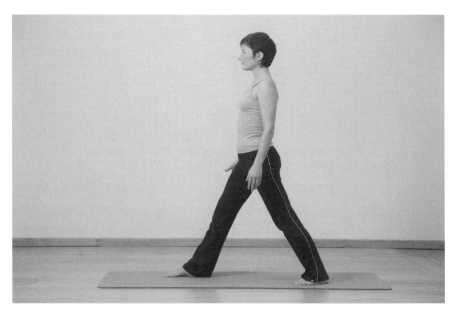

Figure 6.30. Forward Bending Posture

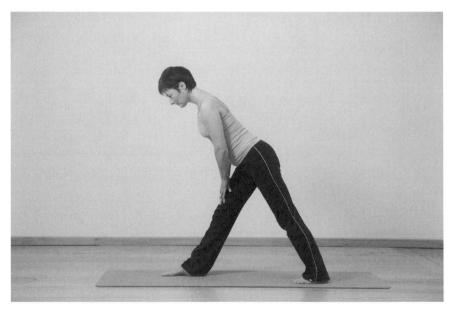

Figure 6.31. Forward Bending Posture

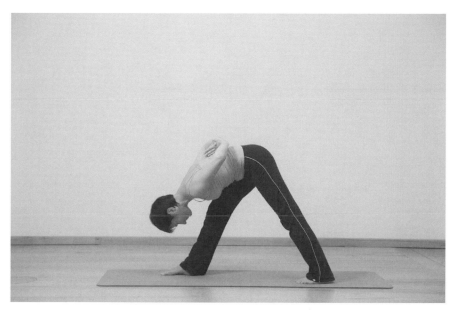

Figure 6.32. Forward Bending Posture

Variation: If you have strong back muscles, good balance, and a flexible spine, bend your upper body further forward. Bring your palms together behind your upper back. Hold this forward bend for six full inhalations and exhalations (Figure 6.32).

Triangle in Motion

- Come into the standing posture (see "basic stances"). Place your feet more than shoulder width apart (Figure 6.33).
- While breathing in through your nose, slowly raise your arms over the sides until they are fully stretched over your head. Only raise your arms;; do not pull up your shoulders. If you are not exactly sure, you may raise your shoulders briefly and let them sink again.
- With your right hand take hold of the wrist of your left hand (Figure 6.34).
- Exhale and stretch your arm with the help of your hand and bend your upper body to the right side. Make sure you do not bend forward. Keep both your arms and flanks stretched. Keep your head and neck straight (Figure 6.35).

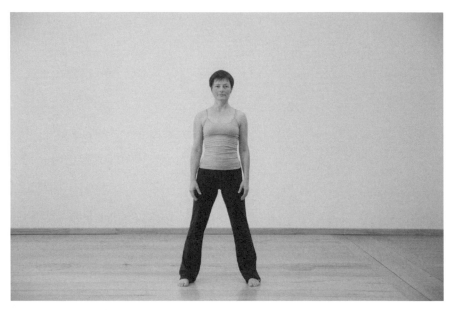

Figure 6.33. Triangle in Motion

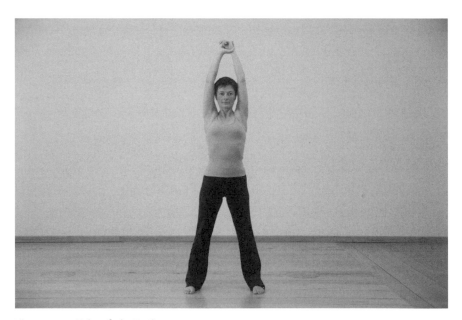

Figure 6.34. Triangle in Motion

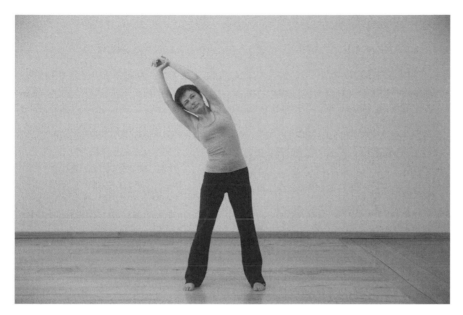

Figure 6.35. Triangle in Motion

- Inhal, return to the upright position, and change the positions of your hands.
- Exhale and bend to the other side.
- Repeat the exercise for six complete inhalations and exhalations.
- Finally, stay in the standing posture and feel the stretches of your flanks. Close your eyes if it is pleasant for you.

Stiff Knees, Tired Legs and Feet: Rotate, Bend, and Lift

Sudden side-to-side movements, as well as long hours with bent knees while seated or blocked knees while standing, may hurt your knees. Poor posture of the knees often accompanies a poor position of the torso. Weak thigh muscles fail to keep the pelvis aligned and put more weight on the knees.

The following rotations of knees support you in finding the proper alignment. The runner posture helps you to build thigh muscles. The palm tree posture brings you up to the tip of your toes, which enhances the circulation in your legs and strengthens your feet muscles.

Knee Rotation

- Come into the standing posture (see "basic stances").
- Bend both your knees and put your hands on top of your kneecaps. Your fingers are facing downward (Figure 6.36).
- Fully stretch out your spine and do not bow your upper torso.
- Slowly rotate your knees in one direction and maintain a regular breathing rhythm (Figure 6.37).
- Continue in this direction while you do six complete inhalations and exhalations.
- Change the direction and do the rotation to the other side during the next six full breath cycles (Figure 6.38).
- Gently stop the movement, roll your body upward with your knees bent, come into the standing posture, and feel the effects in your knees. You may close your eyes if you like.

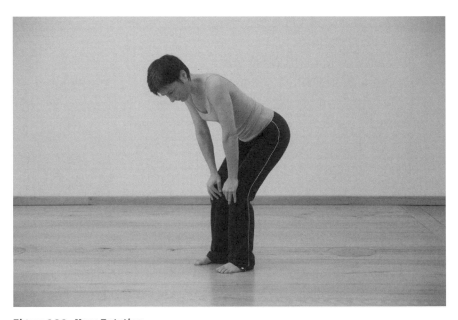

Figure 6.36. Knee Rotation

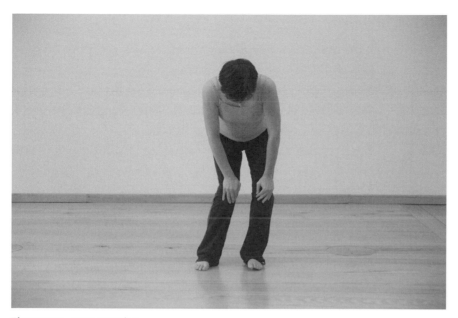

Figure 6.37. Knee Rotation

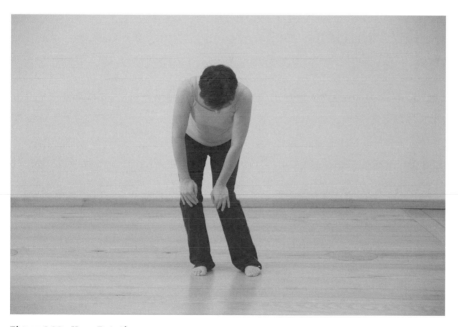

Figure 6.38. Knee Rotation

Runner Posture

- Come into the standing posture (see "basic stances"). Stand in front of a chair or table.
- Put one foot forward. Make sure that your feet are still hip joint width apart and that the outer sides of your feet are parallel. Keep both legs stretched and both heels on the floor.
- With an exhalation, slowly bend your front leg and lower your torso until your hands touch the chair and the knee of your back leg touches the floor. Make sure that your spinal column is fully stretched out and your pelvis muscles are tight. To keep your knees healthy, make sure that your front knee is in line with the front ankle (Figure 6.39).
- Maintain the position for six full inhalations and exhalations.
- While inhaling, lift the knee of your stretched leg and stretch your front knee. Return to the starting position.
- Move your front foot backward and get into the standing posture.
- Close your eyes and compare both sides—both legs, both sides of your pelvis, and both sides of your face.
- Repeat the exercise on the other side.
- Finally, get into the standing posture, close your eyes, and feel the balancing effect of the whole exercise.

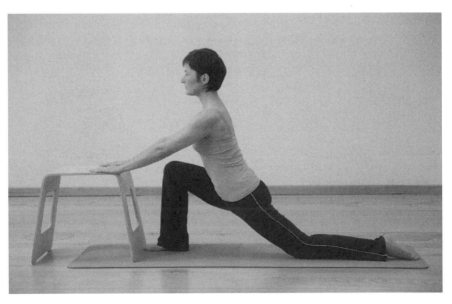

Figure 6.39. Runner Posture

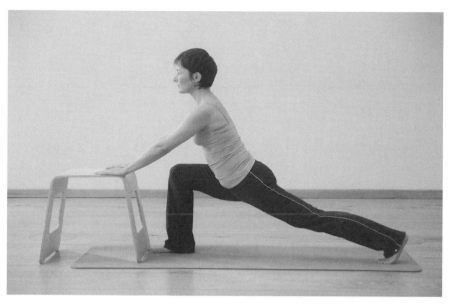

Figure 6.40. Runner Posture

Variation: If you have strong legs, strong back muscles, and good balance, stretch out your leg backward (do not bend your knee and do not let it touch the mat) and push your back heel toward the ground. Hold this posture for six full inhalations and exhalations (Figure 6.40).

Palm Tree Posture

- Come into the standing posture (see "basic stances").
- Inhale and lift your arms sideways, cross your fingers, and place your hands on your head with your palms turned outward (Figure 6.41).
- Breathe in through your nose while stretching your arms and lifting your heels until your weight is balanced on the tips of your toes (Figure 6.42).
- Breathe out through your nose while slowly lowering your arms to your sides (Figure 6.43) and placing your feet on the ground with the weight evenly spread over your soles.
- Repeat the movement during six complete inhalations and exhalations.

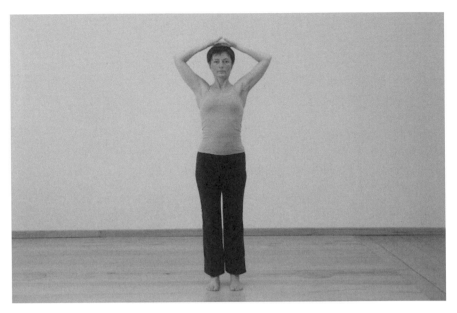

Figure 6.41. Palm Tree Posture

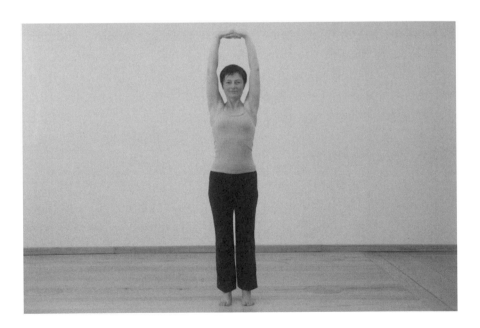

Figure 6.42. Palm Tree Posture

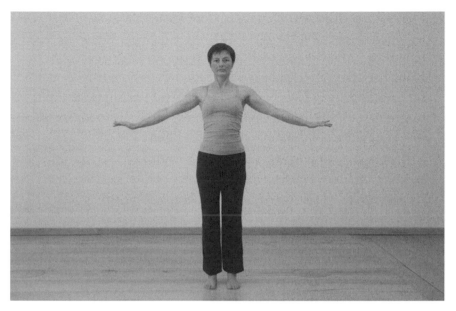

Figure 6.43. Palm Tree Posture

● Finally, return to the standing posture and feel the energy in your
  feet and the effects of the balancing posture. If it is comfortable,
  close your eyes.

Little Energy and Poor Posture: Recharge and Increase Your Strength

Yoga helps strengthen your muscles as well as your nervous system.
You can build up energy with the right breathing techniques and the
right movements. Yoga is a good antidote for loss of energy. Yoga exercises and yoga breathing techniques can boost your circulation.

The following exercises help you to build muscles from your
feet up to your arms. They are demanding but also very energizing.
You can also experience how muscle strength helps you to stay in
balance.

Hero 1 Posture

● Come into the standing posture (see "basic stances").

- Put one foot forward. Make sure that your feet are still hip joint width apart and that the outer sides of your feet are parallel. Keep both legs stretched and both heels on the floor.
- Bring both palms together in front of your sternum (Figure 6.44).
- Inhale and slowly lower your front leg while pushing your elbows backward and stretching your shoulders. Make sure your front knee is properly aligned over your ankle (Figure 6.45).
- Exhale and slowly move back into the starting position with palms together and the front knee stretched.
- Repeat the exercise for six full inhalations and exhalations.
- With an inhalation, return to the starting position.
- Move your front foot backward and get into the standing posture.
- Close your eyes and compare both sides—both legs, both sides of your pelvis, and both sides of your face.
- Repeat the exercise on the other side.
- Finally, get into the standing posture, close your eyes, and feel the stretch of your back and the balancing effect of the whole exercise.

Variation: If you have good balance, stretch out your arms and look upward. Hold this posture for six full inhalations and exhalations (Figure 6.46). Make sure your back heel remains in contact with the floor.

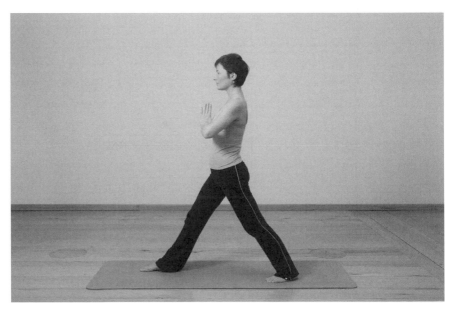

Figure 6.44. Hero 1 Posture

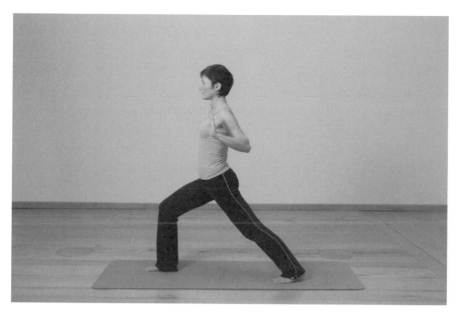

Figure 6.45. Hero 1 Posture

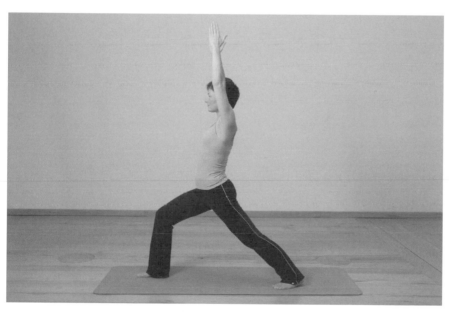

Figure 6.46. Hero 1 Posture

Stargazer Posture

- Come into the standing posture (see "basic stances").
- Put one foot forward. Make sure that your feet are still hip joint width apart and that the outer sides of your feet are parallel. Keep both legs stretched and both heels on the floor (Figure 6.47).
- Bring both palms together behind your back. [If you do not yet have the flexibility, bring your hands to your elbows] (Figure 6.48).
- With an inhalation, stretch your spinal column and look upward. Make sure your pelvis muscles are tight.
- Maintain the position for six full inhalations and exhalations.
- With an inhalation, return to the starting position.
- Move your front foot backward and get into the standing posture.
- Close your eyes and compare both sides—both legs, both sides of your pelvis, and both sides of your face.
- Repeat the exercise on the other side.
- Finally, get into the standing posture, close your eyes, and feel the effect of the whole exercise.

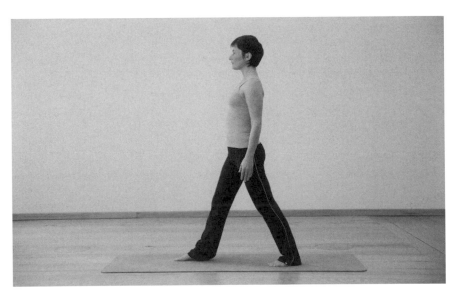

Figure 6.47. Stargazer Posture

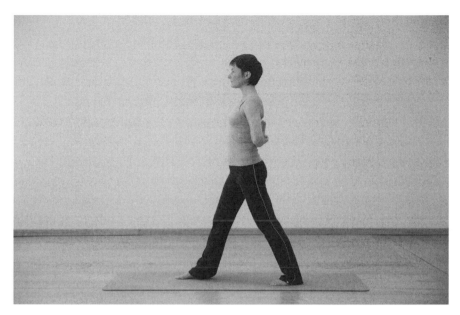

Figure 6.48. Stargazer Posture

Variation: If you have good balance and a flexible spine, bend your upper body further backward. Hold this backward bend for six full inhalations and exhalations.

Moody and Feeling Blue: Lift Your Spirit

There are times when you feel moody or blue. To help you out of this mood, to ease any soreness, and to calm your mind, you need yoga asana that are energizing and balancing.

In particular, the hero postures are good for this purpose. They strengthen your leg muscles and help you obtain good posture. At the same time, you will be regaining your standing position and feel more confident.

Bend and Twist

- Come into the standing posture (see "basic stances").

- Position your feet one leg length apart. Make sure both soles and both outer sides of your feet are touching the ground. Bend your knees.
- Inhale and stretch out your spine.
- Exhale while slowly bending your torso down until the tips of your fingers touch the floor. Stretch your knees. Make sure your back is stretched out. If not, put a thick book (two books) or a little stool in front of you (Figure 6.49).
- Put one hand into the middle underneath your chest and turn it outward.
- Inhale while slowly raising the free hand over the side and upward. You feel the twist in your upper vertebrae. Stretch out both arms with the lower hand pushing the ground and the upper hand stretched out toward the ceiling (Figure 6.50).
- If you have a flexible neck, turn your head and look upward toward your upper hand.
- Exhale while slowly moving back. Change the position of your hands.
- Inhale and do the exercise on the other side.
- Finally, stay in the forward bending posture with fingertips on the ground.
- Bend your knees, inhale, and slowly roll your torso upward.
- Bring your feet closer together and return to the standing posture. Feel the effects of the exercise. Close your eyes if you like.

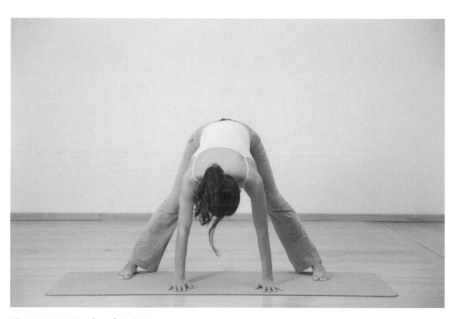

Figure 6.49. Bend and Twist

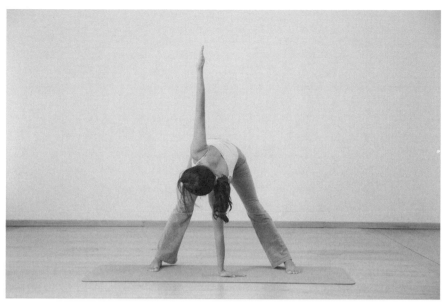

Figure 6.50. Bend and Twist

Hero 2 Posture

- Come into the standing posture see "basic stances").
- Turn one foot completely outward and take a step forward into the same direction.
- Turn the other foot 45 degrees inward. Make sure that your pelvis is in the same position as it was when you started (Figure 6.51).
- Inhale slowly, raising your arms up to shoulder height. Stretch out both arms and keep the stretch. Feel it in your arms and in your fingertips.
- Exhale and slowly bend the front knee forward until it is at the same height as the ankle of your front foot.
- Turn your head and look over the stretched out side. Make sure that your torso is in an upright position, and do not bend forward (Figure 6.52).
- Keep the position for six full inhalations and exhalations.
- With an inhalation, stretch both legs and lower your arms.
- Bring your feet closer together and compare both sides of your body: both legs, both sides of your pelvis, both shoulders, and both sides of your face.
- Repeat the posture on the other side.

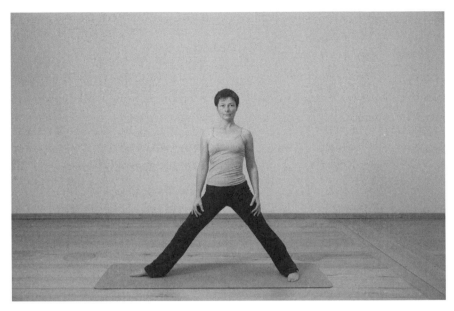

Figure 6.51. Hero 2 Posture

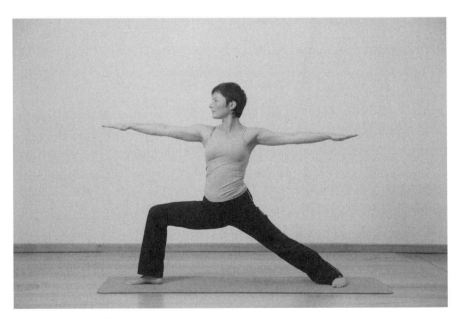

Figure 6.52. Hero 2 Posture

- Finally, return to the standing posture and feel the energy in your body. Close your eyes if you like.

Low Concentration: Improve Memory and Stay Focused

A high-energy level and a good mental focus are essential for health professionals. Yoga enhances our ability to physically and mentally rise to the challenges of our jobs.

The following exercises help you become focused and balanced. They also improve your respiration and increase your circulation. More oxygen is transported with the blood.

Tree Posture

- Come into the standing posture (see "basic stances").
- Shift your weight to your left leg.
- While inhaling, bend your right leg—the one not holding your weight —and push the soles of your right foot against the inner side of your inner left ankle. Rotate your bent leg outward as far as possible (Figure 6.53).
- Bring your palms together in front of your sternum. Relax your shoulders, your face muscles, your lips, and your tongue.
- Maintain this posture for six complete inhalations and exhalations.
- With an inhalation, rotate your bent leg inward, lift it up, and hold it in front of the right side of your chest with both your hands.
- While exhaling, take hold of your knee with both your hands and move it toward your body.
- With an inhalation, loosen your fingers.
- Finally, with the next exhalation, slowly lower your bent leg, stretch it out, and place it on the ground.
- Close your eyes and compare both sides of your body: left and right leg, left and right side of your pelvis, and left and right side of your face.
- Repeat the exercise on the other side.
- Finally, return to the standing posture and again feel both sides of the body. Close your eyes if it feels comfortable.

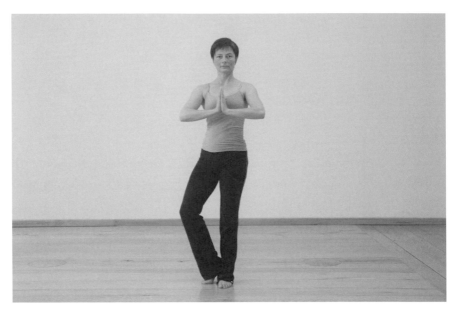

Figure 6.53. Tree Posture

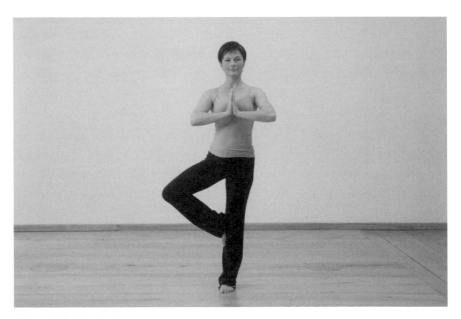

Figure 6.54. Tree Posture

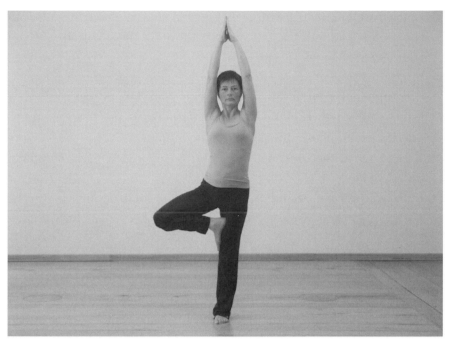

Figure 6.55. Tree Posture

Variation: If you have enough strength in your feet and legs and a good sense of balance, you can place your sole either on the inner side of your knee (Figure 6.54) or higher on the inner side of your thigh with arms stretched upward (Figure 6.55).

Alternate Nostril Breathing

- Come into the seated posture on a chair (see "basic stances").
- Bend the index finger, middle finger, and ring finger of your left hand and stretch out your thumb and little finger.
- Place your thumb next to your left nostril and your little finger next to the right nostril. Either place your bent arm on the table or hold it comfortably in front of your body in such a way that it is not pushing on your thorax and is not blocking your breathing.
- To begin, first breathe out deeply through both nostrils.
- Then close your left nostril with your thumb and slowly breathe in through your right nostril. Maintain the position and feel your filled lungs (Figure 6.56).

- Close the right nostril with your little finger and slowly breathe out completely through the left nostril. Maintain the position and feel your "empty" lungs (Figure 6.57).
- Slowly breathe in again through the left nostril. Maintain the position and feel your filled lungs. Close your left nostril with your thumb and slowly breathe out through the right nostril again. Maintain the position and feel your "empty" lungs.
- Repeat the alternate nostril breathing for at least six complete breath cycles.
- Finally, lower your hand and breathe in and out through both your nostrils. Feel the calming effects. Keep your eyes closed if you like.

Variation: To achieve as even a breathing rhythm as possible, you can count to six between every inhalation and every exhalation and to three during the breaks in-between. Your volume of breath can be increased with time. After doing this exercise for some time, you can perform the exercises at a ratio of 8:4, 10:5, and more. This depends, however, on your ability to achieve a pleasant, thorough, and even breathing rhythm.

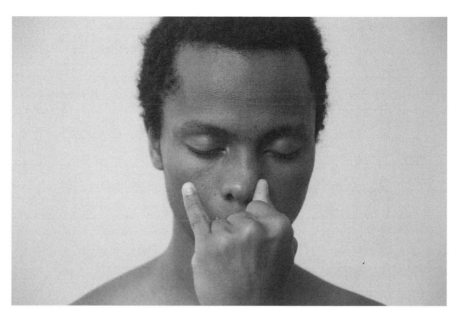

Figure 6.56. Alternate Nostril Breathing

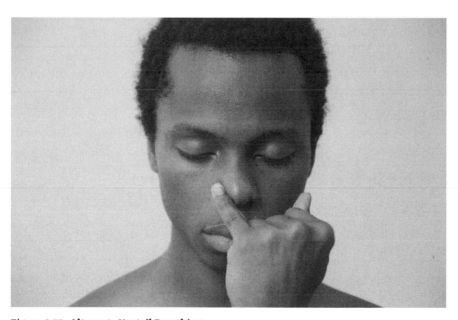

Figure 6.57. Alternate Nostril Breathing

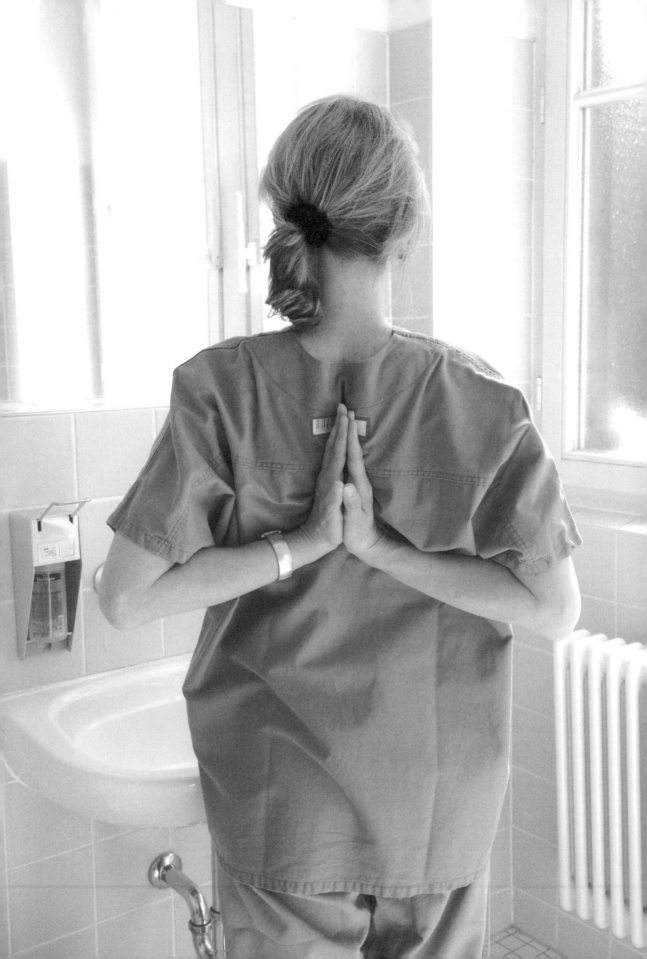

Yoga
Exercises
at Home

7

This chapter presents an attractive variety of yoga postures performed in motion or held in silence to let you enjoy your yoga practice. Though these asana encompass a large variety of exercises, they are all easy do-able in their basic mode. You should continue with the basic mode until you are aware of the effects these asana have on your body and mind. More challenging variations can be considered if you have practiced for a longer time and if you know what an advanced version can do for you. All asana are precisely described and serve the needs of people who want to soothe, cure, or prevent back problems and who want to be more focused and better equipped to relieve work stress.

Remember to do the following:

- Wear comfortable clothes such as pants and t-shirts that feel good and sit well. Practice yoga with bare feet whenever you can.
- Use a nonslip yoga mat or exercise on the floor and use a blanket for all relaxing, breathing, and concentrating exercises. Roll up your blanket and use it as a bolster for your knees or as a support for your head—if you like or need it.
- Inhale and exhale through your nose. There are only a few exceptions in the following exercises, and these are marked.
- Maintain your breathing rhythm while practicing yoga. At the beginning practice with six complete inhalations and exhalations; this is equal to six complete movements.
- Keep your eyes open. At the end of an exercise or after you have worked on one side of the body, you may close your eyes if it helps you to feel the effects. After some practice, you might prefer to exercise with your eyes closed.
- Always start the exercises on the same side of the body.
- If possible, practice at the same place and at the same time; watch your improvements and become aware of your current strengths and weaknesses.
- You will always feel better once you get going.

If you suffer from pain in your back or from work stress, you should practice yoga regularly at work as well as at home. A steady yoga practice is one of the best means of relieving pain and stress. Some yoga asana are easy to do and are very effective. They are very suitable for beginners and are "classics" for experienced yoga students. In this chapter, they are depicted under the title of "core asana."

To help you develop an individual practice, more asana with comparable effects are presented under the heading of "Elective Asana." You can select your favorite posture or you can try out different postures each day within each section.

- Awareness and alignment
- Breathing techniques, body exercises, and balancing asana
- Relaxing and awareness

Opening Section	Self Awareness and Supine Postures
Main Section	Pranayama Dynamic Asana Realign Again
Closing Section	Relax and Become Aware of the Effects

Enjoying Yourself Doing Yoga:
A Suitable Program for Yoga at Home

The left column of the box details the asana you should practice regularly: core asana. If you practice each asana for six complete inhalations and exhalations, you will need 15 to 30 minutes to complete these core asana. At the beginning, you will need extra time for reading, practicing, and reaffirming these asana.

The right column of the box details the asana you can add to your practice—depending on your special needs. For example, if you have pain in the lower part of your vertebrae and pelvis and need more asana to support your posture and help you realign, you can try out elective asana such as hip rotation, leg lift, and ventral arm and leg stretch.

All Postures at a Glance

Basic Stances for Yoga Exercises at Home	
Core Asana	**Elective Asana**
Lying on the Back	
Kneeling Posture	
Upright Seated Posture	
Free Seat	Half Lotus Seat
	Complete Lotus Seat

Self Awareness and Supine Postures	
Core Asana	**Elective Asana**
Shanti Asana Posture (Awareness)	
Tree Posture on the Floor (Opening Stretch)	
Easy Crocodile Posture (Lower Back and Pelvis)	Hip Rotation (Hip Joints)
	Leg Lift Sideways (Hip Joints, Pelvis and Leg Muscles)
Knee to Chest (Lower Back and Knees)	
Dorsal Arms and Legs Stretch (Shoulder, Back, and Belly)	Ventral Arms and Legs Stretch (Dorsal Strength)
	Cobra Posture/Sphinx Posture (Dorsal Strength)
	Spider Posture (Counterstretching after Back Bends)

Pranayama, Dynamic Asana, and Realign Again	
Core Asana	**Elective Asana**
Detox Breathing (Tension Relief and Thorough Breathing) Variation: Folded Leaf (Neck and Back Stretch)	Camel Posture (Thigh Muscles and Lower Breathing Space)
	Great Gesture (Neck and Shoulder Muscles and Upper Breathing Space)
Tiger Breathing (Synchronization of Breathing and Moving)	Alternate Nostril Breathing (Expands the Breathing Capacity, Calms, and Helps Concentration)

Pranayama, Dynamic Asana, and Realign Again (continued)	
Core Asana	**Elective Asana**
	Table Posture (Arm, Leg, and Belly Muscles and Breathing Space)
	Fish Posture (Neck, Shoulder, Back, Rib Cage, and Upper Breathing Space)
Sunbird (Combination of Three Asana)	Threading the Needle (Shoulders and Upper Torso)
Child Posture (Arm and Back Stretch and Strength)	Runner Posture (Leg and Spine Stretch)
Tiger Posture (Back Bow and Stretch)	Pyramid Posture (Leg and Spine Stretch)
	Triangle Posture (Stretches the Flanks)
Mountain Posture (Arm, Back, and Leg Stretch and Strength)	Boat Posture (Abdominal Strength)
Shoulder Bridge (Flexibility and Strength of Back and Leg Muscles)	Cow Posture (Neck, Shoulders, and Arms)
Crocodile Posture (Flexibility and Strength of Belly Muscles)	
Relax and Become Aware of the Effects	
Core Asana	**Elective Asana**
Shanti Asana (Complete Relaxation and Deepening of the Effects)	
Free Seat or Kneeling Posture (Stabilizing the Blood Circulation and Awareness of the Effects	Half Lotus or Complete Lotus Posture (Stabilizing the Blood Circulation, Awareness of the Effects, and Special Stretch of Legs and Hips)

Basic Stances for Yoga Exercises at Home

Basic stances exist when you are stretched out on the floor—lying on your back, belly, chest, or side. Seated basic stances are either done on the floor or on a chair—challenging the muscles and joints of the legs, knees, and feet differently, but always with the weight of the body evenly distributed on the sit bones. Standing basic stances are generally done with the feet on the floor and with the weight evenly distributed on the soles of the feet—but also on the shoulders, forearms, hands, or head.

Their Purposes

Basic stances occur at the beginning of the exercise time or of a single posture. They are a definite part of each posture and allow you to recognize the difference before and after you have exercised. Basic stances also occur during the asana. After finishing half of the asana, you remain in the basic stance, allowing you to recognize the differences between the upper and lower part, left and right side, and front and back side of the body. This allows you to recognize your polarity.

The more often you have been in a basic stance, the better you are able to recognize your definite body tone, your actual breathing rhythm, and the depth of your breathing and the more you become aware of your thoughts and feelings. Proper basic stances enhance your general posture, deepen your breathing, and support your ability to become focused.

Last, but not least, basic stances are an essential part of breathing, concentrating, and meditating postures. The better you manage these postures the longer you can practice the various techniques.

Contraindications

There are no contraindications to the basic stances. However, some of the basic stances can be difficult on your knees. If it is difficult for you to kneel on your heels, use a bolster (folded blanket) as a prop and put it under your knees or under your stretched feet. If you have problems bending your legs and knees to come into the half lotus seat or complete lotus seat, be aware of the reasons for the problems. If you have knee problems you should not do these seats. If you lack the flexibility to do the positions, you can improve your ability step by step by using cushions as bolsters in the beginning.

People with uncontrolled high blood pressure and eye and ear conditions should keep their heads above heart level and rest on a cushion or folded blanket. Jumping up suddenly from a calm stance might lead to a decrease in blood pressure and make people feel dizzy. Slowly inhale while rolling upward into a standing posture or while gently moving into the next asana.

Alignment

In all the basic stances the spinal column is stretched out between the pelvis and head crown, the sternum is raised, and shoulders and arms as well as the face and tongue muscles are relaxed. The breath flows in and out through the nose.

Core Asana

Lying on Your Back

- Relax your entire body while lying on your back.
- Your arms lie on the sides of your body with the palms facing downward.
- Your neck is stretched.
- Your face and mouth muscles are relaxed (Figure 7.1).

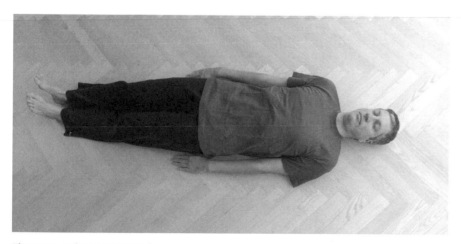

Figure 7.1. Lying on Your Back

- Completely breathe in and out through your nose.
- Close your eyes if it feels comfortable.

Variation. Place your head on a folded blanket or cushion if you have uncontrolled high blood pressure or ear and eye conditions.

Kneeling Posture

- Distribute your sit bones on your heels. Your feet are stretched and tipped neither inwardly nor outwardly.
- Your pelvis is upright, your bottom, or rather your pelvis muscles, are tight, and your belly is relaxed.
- Your spinal column is straightened, and your sternum is raised.
- Your shoulders and arms are relaxed, and your hands are resting on your thighs or on the floor (Figure 7.2).
- Your face and mouth muscles are relaxed.
- Completely breathe in and out through your nose.

Variation: If the posture feels uncomfortable, use a cushion or a folded blanket. Make sure that you use the bolster in the right place. At first place the cushion under your knees and determine the effect. Then

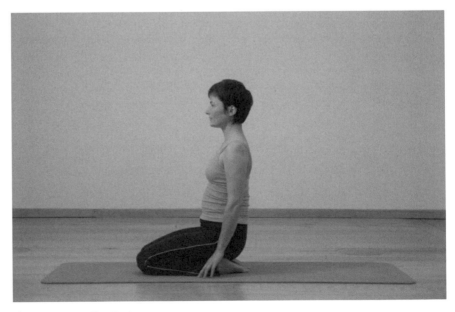

Figure 7.2. Kneeling Posture

place the cushion under your ankles and feet and determine the effect. Decide in which position the cushion better serves your needs.

Upright Seated Posture

- Take a seat on the floor, and distribute your weight evenly on both sit bones.
- Position your feet hip joint width apart from one another and bend your feet (pull your toes and feet in the direction of your belly).
- Your pelvis is upright, the entire length of your spinal column is stretched, and your head crown extends upward.
- Your sternum is raised, and your hands lay loosely on your thighs.
- Your chin is parallel to the ground, and your face, lips, and tongue are relaxed (Figure 7.3).
- Completely breathe in and out through your nose.

Variation: If your back tends to bend forward, place both hands on the floor behind you to support your upright posture.

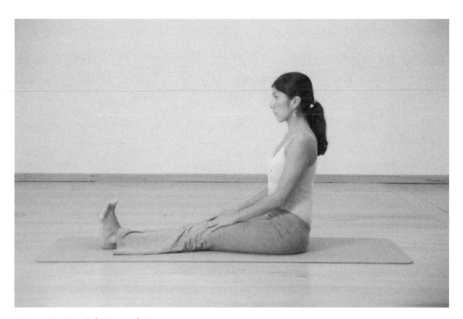

Figure 7.3. Upright Seated Posture

Free Seat

- Take a seat on the floor, and distribute your weight evenly on both sit bones.
- Bend your left knee, and place your left foot in front of your pubic bone.
- Bend your right knee, and place your right foot in front of your left foot.
- Your hands or forearms rest on your knees and thighs. [The model shows a hand gesture called Cin Mudra (seal of awareness). This is an often shown gesture. Bring the tips of your thumb and index finger together, forming a circle.]
- Your pelvis is upright, the entire length of your spinal column is stretched, and your head crown extends upward.
- Your sternum is raised, and your belly is relaxed.
- Your chin is parallel to the ground, and your face, lips, and tongue are relaxed (Figure 7.4).
- Completely breathe in and out through your nose.
- Close your eyes if you like.

Variation: If the free seat does not feel comfortable sit on a folded blanket or cushion.

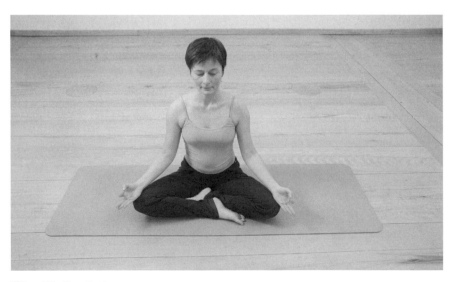

Figure 7.4. Free Seat

Elective Asana

Half Lotus Seat

- Take a seat on the floor, and distribute your weight evenly on both sit bones.
- Bend your left knee, and place your left foot in front of your pubic bone.
- Bend your right leg, and take hold of your right knee and right foot and place them on top of your left thigh near the hip crease.
- Your hands or forearms rest on your knees and thighs.
- Your pelvis is upright, the entire length of your spinal column is stretched, and your head crown extends upward.
- Your sternum is raised, and your belly is relaxed.
- Your chin is parallel to the ground, and your face, lips, and tongue are relaxed (Figure 7.5).
- Completely breathe in and out through your nose.
- Close your eyes if you like.

Complete Lotus Seat

- Take a seat on the floor and distribute your weight evenly on both sit bones.

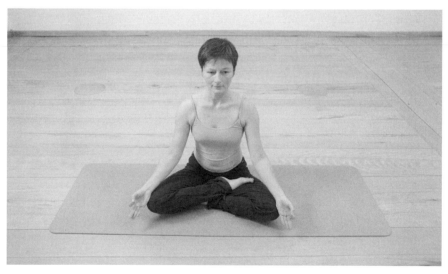

Figure 7.5. Half Lotus Seat

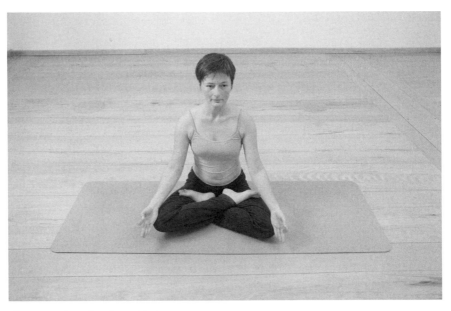

Figure 7.6. Complete Lotus Seat

- Bend your left leg and take hold of your left knee and left foot and place them on top of your right thigh near the hip crease.
- Bend your right leg and take hold of your right knee and right foot and place them on top of your left thigh near the hip crease.
- Your hands or forearms rest on your knees and thighs.
- Your pelvis is upright, the entire length of your spinal column is stretched, and your head crown extends upward (Figure 7.6).
- Your sternum is raised, and your belly is relaxed.
- Your chin is parallel to the ground, and your face, lips, and tongue are relaxed.
- Completely breathe in and out through your nose.
- Close your eyes if you like.

Self Awareness

Shanti asana marks the beginning of our exercises at home. It is one of the basic stances and is done in a stretched out manner on the floor lying on your back.

The more often you have been in shanti asana, the better you are able to recognize your actual body tone, your actual breathing rhythm, and the depth of your breathing; you also become more aware of your thoughts and feelings. Shanti asana enhances your general posture, deepens your breathing, and aids you in becoming focused.

The tree posture on the floor provides the first stretch. Since it is done on the floor, you can be sure that your complete back is stretched.

Contraindications

There are no contraindications for shanti asana or the tree posture on the ground. People with uncontrolled high blood pressure and eye and ear conditions should keep their heads above heart level and rest on a cushion or folded blanket while doing the postures. Jumping up suddenly out of the postures might lead to a decrease in blood pressure and make you feel dizzy. Slowly inhale while rolling upward into a standing posture or gently move into the following asana.

Alignment

In shanti asana, as well as in the tree posture, the spinal column is stretched out between the pelvis and head crown. Do not forget to stretch your neck. The sternum is raised, and your shoulders as well as your face and tongue muscles are relaxed. The breath flows in and out through the nose.

The following questions can help you check your proper alignment and be more conscious of your whole body: Is my neck stretched? Is my face relaxed? Are my tongue and larynx relaxed? Are both my shoulders and arms lying evenly on the ground? Which parts of my feet and legs are touching the ground? Which parts of my back are in contact with the mat?

Core Asana

Shanti Asana Posture

Purpose: relaxes and enhances awareness. This posture is also called "Corpse Pose."

- Stretch your entire body while lying on your back.
- Both your feet are rotated outward.

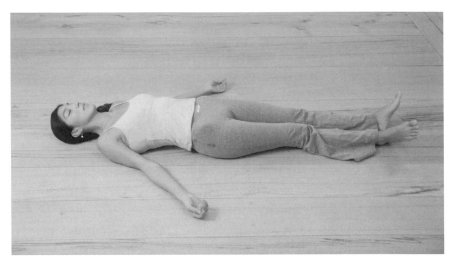

Figure 7.7. Shanti Asana

- Your arms lie on the sides of your body with the palms of the hands facing the ceiling.
- Your shoulders are relaxed and lie on the mat or floor.
- Your neck is stretched.
- Your face and mouth muscles are relaxed.
- Your eyes are closed.
- Completely breathe in and out through your nose.
- Close your eyes if it feels comfortable (Figure 7.7).

Variation: If you suffer from acute pain in your lower back, bend your knees and place your feet on the floor. Keep them more than shoulder width apart and let the inner sides of your knees lean against each other. Fully relax in this position.

Tree Posture on the Floor

Purpose: basic stretch for the whole body; deepens breathing.

- Start from the shanti asana posture (see above). Bend your right leg and place the sole of your right foot against the inner side of your left leg. Your left foot is bent with your toes pointed in the direction of your upper body (Figure 7.8).

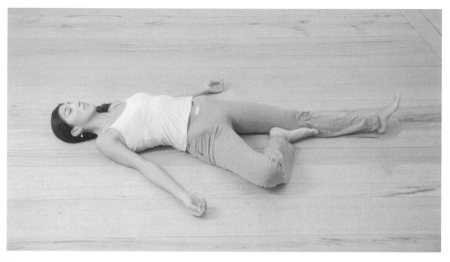

Figure 7.8. Tree Posture on the Floor

- Bring your hands together and cross your fingers. Place your hands on your head with the palms facing upward (away from your head).
- Inhale and stretch your arms and your complete back (Figure 7.9).
- Hold your breath and the stretch for as long as it feels good.
- Slowly exhale through your nose and return to the starting position lowering the arms sideways. Compare the feeling in both sides of

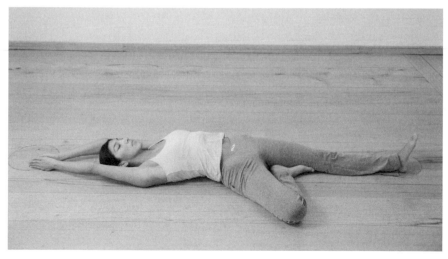

Figure 7.9. Tree Posture on the Floor

your body: both legs and both sides of your pelvis, your shoulders, and your face.

- Repeat the exercise on the other side.
- Finally, get back into the lying posture and feel the effects of the deep breathing and stretching. Close your eyes if you like.

Supine Postures

Supine postures with the following asana are ideal to realign your vertebrae. They are all done stretched out on your back, side, or belly and use the floor as an ideal prop. As long as you can feel the mat or ground against your body, you can be sure you are aligned.

You start with the easy crocodile posture and gentle movements to the sides. If you have serious pain in your lower back, this very small and soothing movement is ideal. It aligns the lower spine and the pelvis. The sacrum or lower end of the vertebrae is connected with the ilium or big pelvis bone through the sacroiliac joint. This is a very delicate joint with little movement but a great ability to block and hurt. Therefore, it is vital to keep this joint flexible. The small movements of the easy crocodile posture serve this purpose.

The knee to chest posture does the same. At the same time, it stretches the lower back toward the belly and creates a lot of space between the vertebrae of the lower back.

You get a good feeling for the flexibility and strength of your muscles when exercising the dorsal leg and arm stretch. The cooperation of the muscles on the back of your legs and back with the muscles of the belly can be felt. Become aware of the mobility of the shoulder joints, as well as the flexibility of the muscles that stretch and bend your arm.

The elected alignments are all very effective. If you have enough time you should do them all. They enhance the mobility of the hip joints in several directions and strengthen the back muscles.

Contraindications

The core alignment postures are easy to do. People with uncontrolled high blood pressure and eye and ear conditions should keep their heads above heart level and rest on a cushion or folded blanket while doing the postures.

The elective asana postures are a little bit more challenging. If you have problems with your hip joints, the hip rotation and the leg lift sideways are ideal. For best results start with small movements and extend them over the time of exercising. People with serious problems in their lower back have to tighten the pelvis muscles and be gentle with the back bends. It is more useful for them to stretch and gain length than to bow and get hurt. For people with uncontrolled high blood pressure and eye and ear conditions, it is important to do the ventral posture with caution because the pressure on the belly vessels may increase the blood pressure.

Alignment

Since all postures are done stretched out on your back, side, or belly with the mat or floor as a prop, it is easy to maintain proper alignment. But be aware: Lying on your side might lead you to bend your upper body forward or to rotate your leg outward, which are not the proper alignments. These issues are addressed in the detailed description of the asana.

Core Asana

Easy Crocodile Posture

Purpose: aligns lower back and pelvis.

- Lie on your back (supine posture), bend your knees, and place both your feet on the mat. Your arms are next to your body and fully relaxed. Your palms are facing downward.
- Slowly bring both your ankles and knees close together (Figure 7.10).
- With the next exhalation, move your knees to one side. Make sure you do small movements only a few inches to the side.
- Inhale and move your knees back into the starting position.
- Exhale and move your knees to the other side.
- Repeat the small movements for at least six complete inhalations and exhalations.

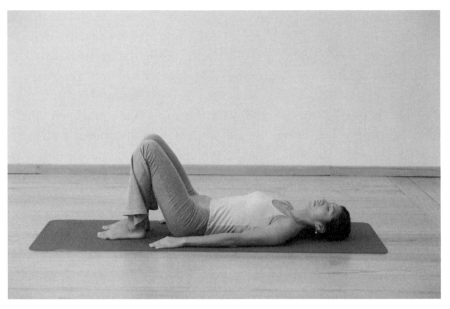

Figure 7.10. Easy Crocodile Posture

● Finally, remain in the starting position and feel the effects of the small movements in your lower back. Close your eyes if it feels comfortable.

Knee to Chest

Purpose: aligns lower back and knees.

● Lie on your back (supine posture), bend both your knees, and place both your feet hip joint width apart on the ground.
● Slowly lift your knees toward your chest and put your left hand on your left knee and your right hand on your right knee. Make sure that both your lower legs and feet are relaxed and that your neck is stretched.
● Exhale through your nose, bend your arms, and pull your knees closer to your chest (Figure 7.11).
● Inhale through your nose, stretch your arms, and bring your knees further away from your chest (Figure 7.12).
● Repeat the movement for six complete inhalations and exhalations.
● Place your feet back on your mat and feel the effects of the movement. Close your eyes if it feels comfortable for you.

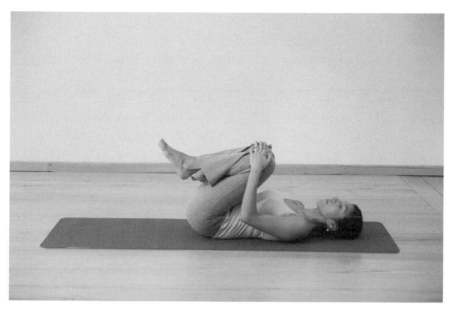

Figure 7.11. Knee to Chest

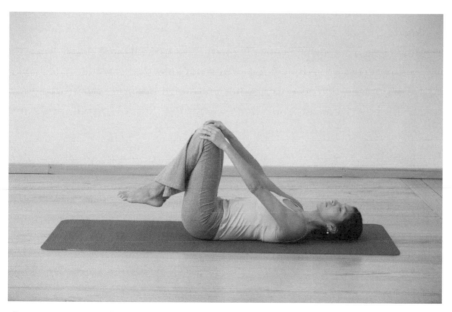

Figure 7.12. Knee to Chest

Variation 1: Extend the exercise by moving your knees in a circle. Exhale while doing the lower half of the circle, and inhale while doing the upper half of the circle. Feel the massage of your lower back.

Variation 2: Do the knee to the chest posture with one knee at a time. Place one foot on the mat and bring the other knee to the chest. Do the knee to the chest posture with one knee. After you have practiced on one side, place both feet on the mat and compare the feeling in your legs, both sides of your pelvis, and both sides of your face. Feel the polarity of your body. Continue to the other side.

Dorsal Arms and Legs Stretch

Purpose: aligns the shoulder and upper back and strengthens the belly muscles.

- Lie on your back (supine posture), bend both your knees, and place both your feet hip joint width apart on the ground. Your arms are stretched out at the side of your body. Both palms are facing downward.
- Lift your knees toward your chest. Make sure that both your lower legs and feet are relaxed and that your neck is stretched (Figure 7.13).
- Inhale while you are stretching your legs upward and lifting your arms. The soles of your feet are facing upward. Your arms are stretched out above your head (Figure 7.14).

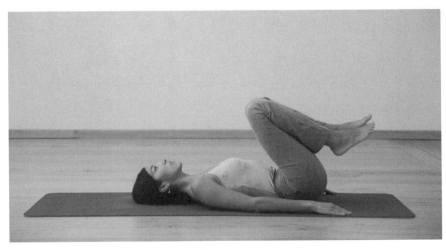

Figure 7.13. Dorsal Arms and Legs Stretch

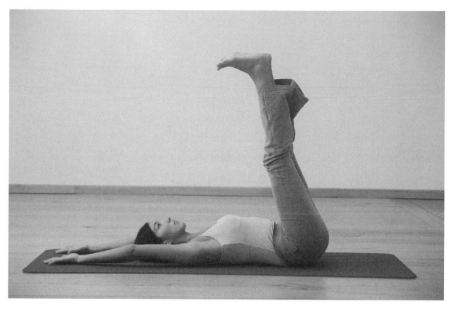

Figure 7.14. Dorsal Arms and Legs Stretch

- Exhale while you are bending your legs and lowering your arms into the starting position.
- Repeat the stretching and bending of legs and arms during six complete inhalations and exhalations.
- Finally, lie on your back and feel the effects of the exercise. You may close your eyes if you like.

Elective Asana

Hip Rotation

Purpose: enhances the flexibility of the hip joints.

- Lie on your back (supine posture), bend both your knees, and place both your feet hip joint width apart on the ground. Your arms are stretched out at the side of your body. Both palms are facing downward. Make sure your neck is stretched and your face and mouth muscles are relaxed (Figure 7.15).
- Inhale while you are stretching out your right leg (Figure 7.16).

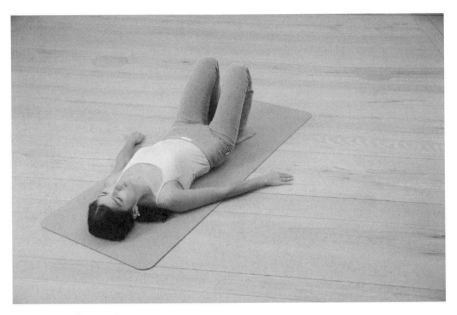

Figure 7.15. Hip Rotation

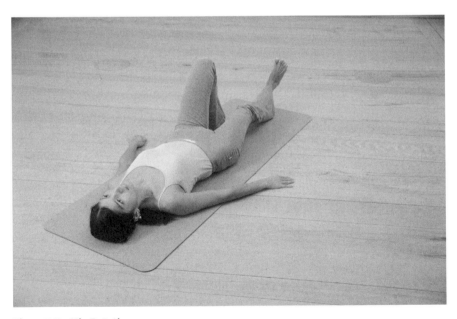

Figure 7.16. Hip Rotation

- Continue the movement doing a circle to the right parallel to the floor (Figure 7.17).
- Exhale while bending your right knee (Figure 7.18) and coming back into the starting position.
- Repeat the movement during six complete inhalations and exhalations.
- Change the direction of the movement on the same side.
- Inhale while rotating your right knee to the right and stretching your right leg and doing a circle.
- Exhale and bend your right leg and bring it back into the starting position.
- Repeat the movement during six complete inhalations and exhalations.
- Place both feet on the ground and compare the feeling in your legs, both sides of your pelvis, and both sides of your face. Feel the polarity of your body.
- Continue to the other side.
- Finally, lie on your back and feel the effects of the complete exercise.

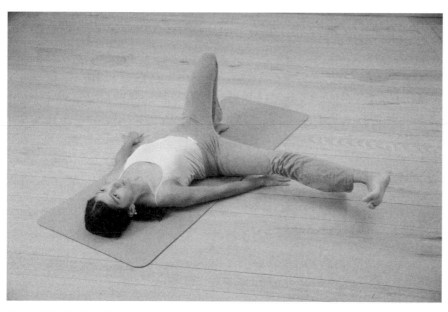

Figure 7.17. Hip Rotation

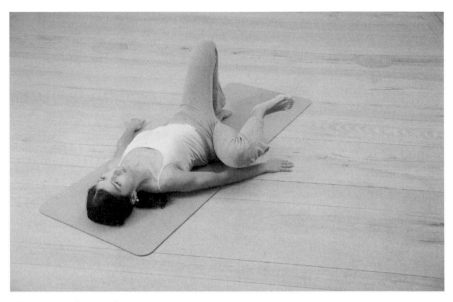

Figure 7.18. Hip Rotation

Leg Lift Sideways

Purpose: enhances the flexibility of the hip joints, aligns vertebrae and pelvis, and strengthens the leg muscles.

- Lie on your back (supine posture), and stretch your right arm.
- Slowly turn to the right side. Make sure that your body is fully stretched out and that you are not bending your upper body. Your feet are bent (toes and feet are pulled toward the belly side).
- Rest your head on your right arm. The left arm is bent and the left hand is placed on the floor in front of your chest. Make sure that you are in a balanced and stable position (Figure 7.19).
- Inhale while you are lifting your upper leg. Make sure you are moving slowly and lifting your leg without rotating your foot (the heel is leading the movement) (Figure 7.20).
- Exhale while you are lowering your upper leg.
- Repeat the movement during six full inhalations and exhalations.
- Turn around on your back and compare the feeling in your legs, both sides of your pelvis, and both sides of your face. Feel the polarity of your body.
- Continue to the other side.
- Finally, lie on your back and feel the effects of the complete exercise.

It is easier to do the exercise if you push your lower leg against the floor while you are lifting your upper leg.

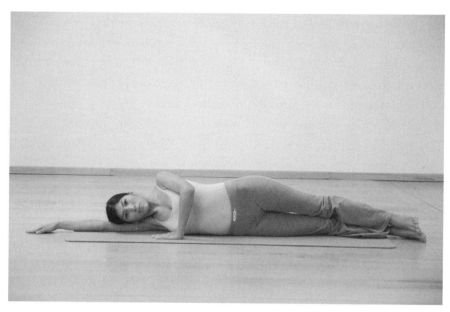

Figure 7.19. **Leg Lift Sideways**

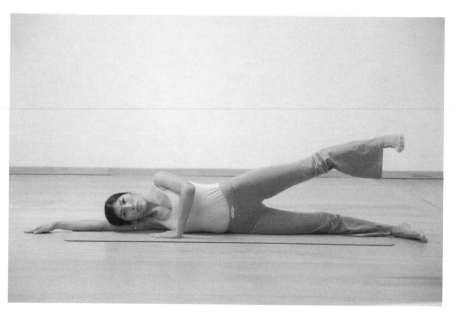

Figure 7.20. **Leg Lift Sideways**

Ventral Arms and Legs Stretch

Purpose: dorsal strength.

- Lie on your back (supine posture), stretch out your left arm, and slowly turn to the left until you are on your stomach.
- Place the front of your body on your mat, and stretch out both arms and legs.
- Tighten your bottom muscles (better your pelvis muscles). Keep these muscles tight during the whole asana.
- Inhale while you are lengthening your right arm and left leg and slowly lift them together with your head. Make sure you are looking downward with your neck stretched out (Figure 7.21).
- Exhale while you are lowering your arm, leg, and head into the starting position.
- Repeat the movement during six full inhalations and exhalations.
- To feel the effects turn your head to the side and rest on your ear. Lower your arms and place them next to your sides, palms facing upward. Your heels are turned outward. Compare both sides of your body.
- Return to the starting position again and repeat the exercise on the other side.

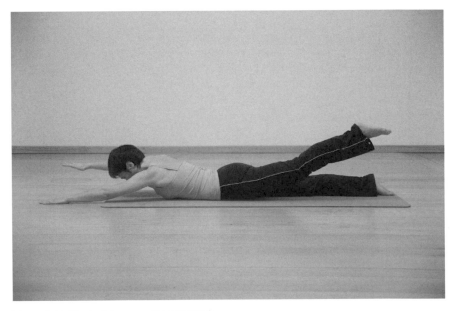

Figure 7.21. Ventral Arms and Legs Stretch

- Turn your head to the other side and rest on your other ear. Lower your arms and place them next to your sides, palms facing upward. Your heels are turned outward. Compare both sides of your body again.
- Finally, turn around again on your back and feel the effects of the whole exercise. Close your eyes if it feels good to you.

Cobra Posture and Sphinx Posture

Purpose: dorsal strength.

- Lie on your back (supine posture), stretch out your left arm, and slowly turn to the left until you are on your stomach.
- Place the front of your body on your mat, bend both your arms, and place your hands next to your shoulders (Figure 7.22).
- Tighten your bottom muscles (that is, your pelvis muscles). Keep these muscles tight during the whole asana.
- Inhale while you are lengthening your spine and slowly lifting it together with your head. Make sure that your neck is stretched out and your shoulders are relaxed (Figure 7.23).
- Exhale while you are lowering your spine and head into the starting position.

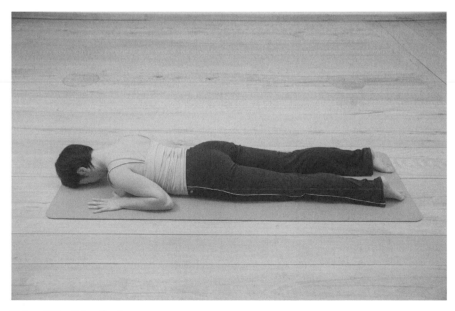

Figure 7.22. Cobra Posture

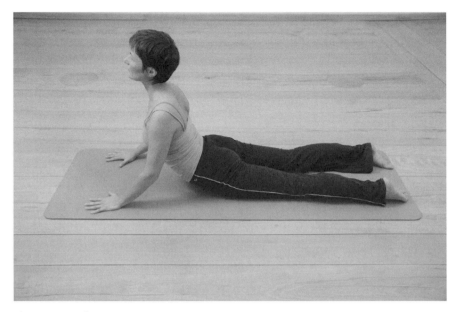

Figure 7.23. Cobra Posture

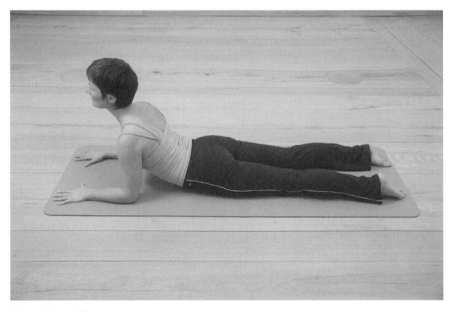

Figure 7.24. Cobra Posture

- Repeat the movement during six full inhalations and exhalations.
- To feel the effects, turn your head to the side and rest on your ear. Lower your arms and place them next to your sides, palms facing upward. Your heels are turned outward.

Variation: Sphinx Posture

- To maintain the posture, place your forearms on the ground while you are lowering your spine and head with an exhalation. Make sure that your elbows are underneath your shoulders (Figure 7.24).
- Maintain the posture for six complete inhalations and exhalations.
- Exhale and return to the starting posture.
- Finally, turn around on your back and feel the effects in this posture. Close your eyes if it feels comfortable for you.

Spider Posture

Purpose: counterstretch after back bends.

- Lie on your back (supine posture), bend both your knees, and place both your feet hip joint width apart on the ground.
- Slowly lift your knees toward your chest.
- Bring your arms between your knees and get hold of your right foot with your right hand and your left foot with your left hand. Lift both lower legs with the help of your hands. Make sure your neck is stretched, your lower back is on the floor, and your thighs are parallel to the floor (Figure 7.25).
- Exhale through your nose and slowly swing your body to your right side (Figure 7.26).
- Inhale through your nose and slowly swing back into the middle.
- Exhale through your nose and slowly swing your body to your left side (Figure 7.27).
- Inhale through your nose and slowly swing back into the middle.
- Repeat the movement for six complete inhalations and exhalations.
- Lower your legs and arms. Place your feet on your mat and your arms at the side of your body.
- Feel the effects of the movement. Close your eyes if it feels comfortable for you.

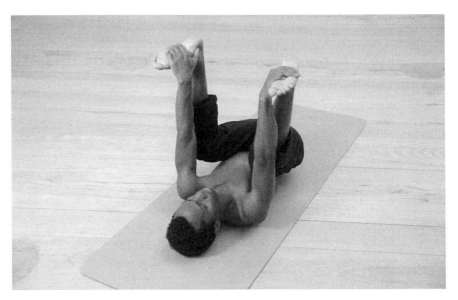

Figure 7.25. Spider Posture

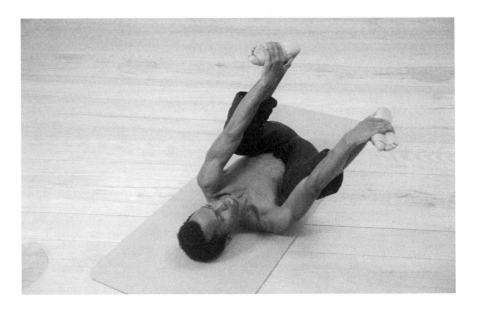

Figure 7.26. Spider Posture

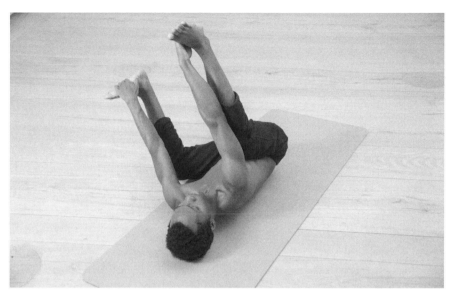

Figure 7.27. Spider Posture

Pranayama

Breathing techniques are always consciously done as a part of an asana or as an exercise in itself: pranayama. They are either done in quiet postures lying or sitting on the floor or parallel with the movements and postures. The synchronizing of breathing and moving is paramount for yoga. Breathing techniques are the companions of all asana. They help us get into postures and to keep the postures.

Breathing techniques are more than just companions when they serve to fuel the circulation or the digestion. They tell you about the actual condition of your body.

Breathing techniques hold a core position when they help you to get focused, to concentrate, and to meditate.

Pranayama exercises influence the diverse sections of the breathing apparatus, that is, the camel posture has greater influence on the diaphragm and deep breathing and the fish posture extends the rip cage and can be felt up to the tips of the lungs, lifting the collarbones.

Their Purposes

To influence our physical and mental well-being via breathing is an essential goal in yoga. The breathing techniques, which are therefore a very important part of yoga, are assembled under one title: pranayama.

You gain strength and self-awareness if you are able to concentrate on your breathing and moving and what it does for you. To be fully concentrated is a good feeling. Therefore, breathing is always consciously done as a part of an asana or as an exercise in itself. It takes considerable practice before you are sure about the movements and you become aware of the breathing and its effects on you.

To inhale and exhale consciously while making small movements is an appropriate way to better focus and concentrate. If you can influence your posture as well as your mind via breathing, it not only helps you to do a satisfactory yoga but also to better manage your workload—physically and mentally. It is crucial to be able to consciously exhale and relax your shoulders and relieve tension or to inhale and lift a weight.

Breathing techniques increase the oxygen level in the blood. The circulation of oxygen-rich blood increases your muscle power as well as your mental power. Pranayama helps to relieve inner tensions and enables you to mentally relax. It can also stimulate the digestion.

Contraindications

There are no contraindications, but it is vital that you do not underestimate the effects of them. If ever you feel faint or nauseated while practicing pranayama, immediately stop the exercise and return to your normal breathing.

Alignment

Regular breathing in yoga is breathing through the nostrils. Exceptions will be marked in this book. The breath initializes and leads the movement. The movement should be completed with an inhalation or with an exhalation. If you feel short of breath slow the movement down.

Core Asana

Detox Breathing

Purpose: tension relief and thorough breathing.

- Come into a kneeling posture (see "basic stances for Yoga at home").
- Place your hands on top of your thighs.
- Inhale through your nose in this position.
- Purse your lips, keep your teeth clenched. Exhale through your mouth (note!) and make the sound "shh." Gently bend downward and exhale more and more each time with a "shh" until your torso is parallel to the ground. Make sure that you do not inhale inbetween (Figure 7.28).
- Inhale, stretch out your neck, and raise your stretched out torso until you are back into the starting position.
- Repeat the forward bend three times.
- After the third time, maintain the position and place your head in front of your knees ("nose between your knees"). Your arms are lying at the side of your body with your palms facing upward (Figure 7.29).

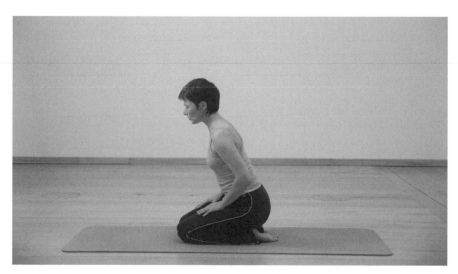

Figure 7.28. Detox Breathing

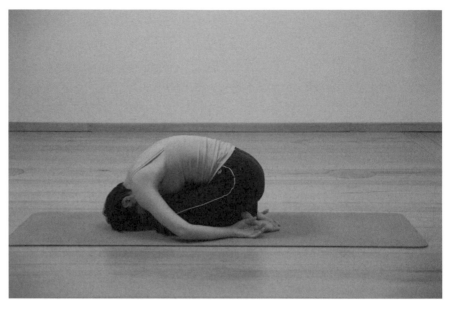

Figure 7.29. Detox Breathing

- Maintain the position for three complete inhalations (feel the stretch of your spine with each inhalation) and three complete exhalations (relax your shoulders with every exhalation).

Note: You can do this position not only in the context of the detox breathing posture. It is a posture in itself, called the folded leaf posture. If you need a break and want to stretch your back or relax your shoulder, get into this posture.

- Gently stretch out your neck.
- Inhale while you are slowly lifting your stretched out torso.
- Place your hands behind your feet. Your fingers are pointing in the direction of your heels. Bend backward and stay in this position. Make sure your sternum is lifted (Figure 7.30).
- Maintain the position for three complete inhalations and exhalations.
- Inhale while you are slowly lifting your stretched out torso.
- Maintain the kneeling posture, place your hands on your thighs, and feel the effects of the whole exercise. Close your eyes if you like.

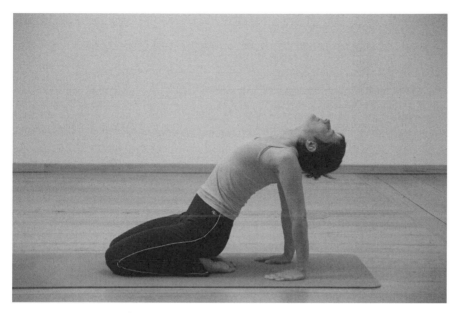

Figure 7.30. Detox Breathing

Variation 1: If you have enough flexibility to bend further backward, you can place your forearms behind you on the ground. Make sure that your knees are close together and still resting on the floor (Figure 7.31).

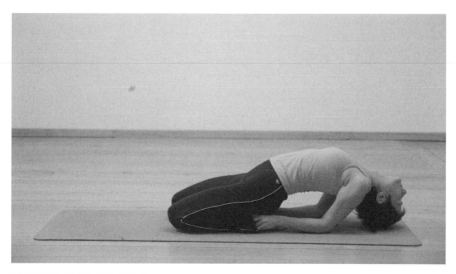

Figure 7.31. Detox Breathing

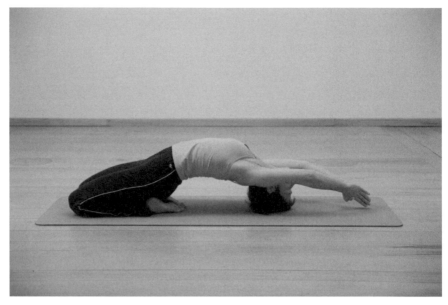

Figure 7.32. Detox Breathing

Variation 2: To put your head on the ground and stretch both arms while doing variation 1, you need great flexibility. Make sure that your knees are close together and still resting on the floor (Figure 7.32).

Tiger Breathing

Purpose: synchronization of breathing and moving.

- Come into the kneeling posture (see "basic stances for Yoga at home").
- With an inhalation, bend forward until your hands touch the floor.
- Make sure that your wrists are under your shoulders and that your knees are under your hip joints. These alignments help you to exercise without hurting your joints.
- Exhale while you are bending your spine vertebra by vertebra starting at your tailbone and moving all the way up: lumbar, thoracic, and cervical spine. Bow your head at the last moment (Figure 7.33).
- Inhale and stretch your spine vertebra by vertebra starting at your tailbone and moving all the way up: lumbar, thoracic, and cervical spine. Lift your head at the last moment (Figure 7.34).

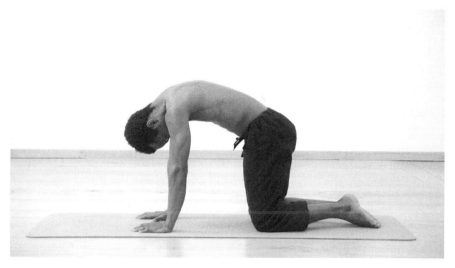

Figure 7.33. Tiger Breathing

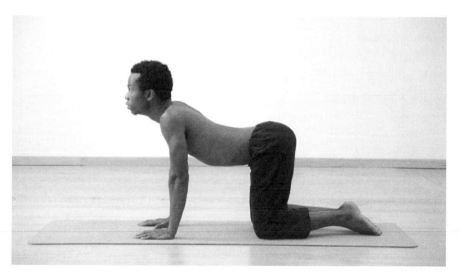

Figure 7.34. Tiger Breathing

- Repeat the bend and stretch for six complete inhalations and exhalations.
- Inhale and return into the kneeling posture again. Place your fingers on top of your thighs and relax. Feel the effects with your eyes closed if you like.

Elective Asana

Camel Posture

Purpose: strengthens thigh and belly muscles, flexes the back, and expands the lower breathing space.

- Come into the kneeling posture (see "basic stances for Yoga at home"), with arms at the side.
- Inhale while rising on your knees, bending your toes, and opening your arms to the side. Make sure your thighs are in an upright position, your pubic bone is pushing forward, and your pelvis muscles are tightened (Figure 7.35).
- Exhale and return to the starting position.
- Repeat the movement for six complete inhalations and exhalations.
- To keep the posture come into the camel posture, place your hands on the lower back, fingers pointing downward and thumbs pointing outward, and maintain the posture for three complete inhalations and exhalations (Figure 7.36).
- With an exhalation, return to the kneeling posture and feel the effects of the exercise.

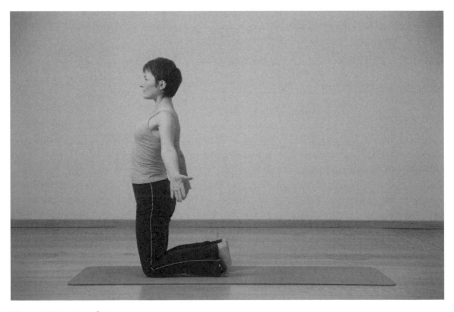

Figure 7.35. Camel Posture

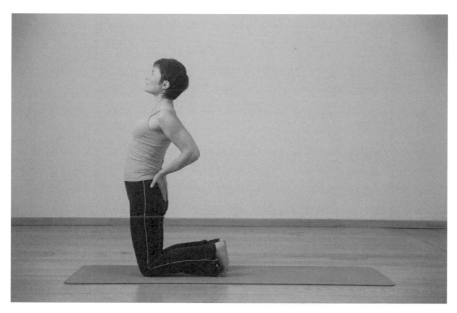

Figure 7.36. Camel Posture

Variation 1: If you have enough flexibility to bend further backward, you can place your hands on your heels. With an inhalation you are rising to your knees simultaneously doing a backward circle with your arms (one after the other). Maintain the position for six complete inhalations and exhalations (Figure 7.37).

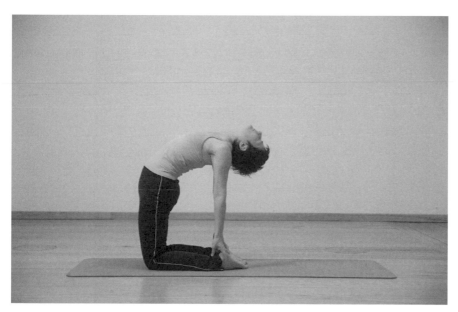

Figure 7.37. Camel Posture

Great Gesture

Purpose: flexes neck and shoulder muscles and enlarges the upper breathing space.

- Come into the kneeling posture (see "basic stances for Yoga at home").
- Stretch out your arms and move them backward. Bring your hands together behind your back and cross your fingers; the palms are facing toward your back (Figure 7.38).
- Inhale through your nose in this position.
- Exhale through your nose while slowly bending your torso forward.
- Place your head on the mat in front of your knees (nose "between your knees") (Figure 7.39).
- Further exhale simultaneously raising and lowering your arms three times (Figure 7.40). (Make sure that you do not inhale in-between and that you use the movement of your arms to entirely exhale.)
- Gently stretch out your neck.
- Inhale while you are slowly lifting your stretched out torso back into the starting position.
- Repeat the movements for six complete inhalations and exhalations.

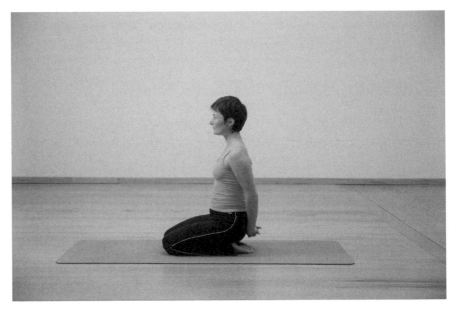

Figure 7.38. Great Gesture

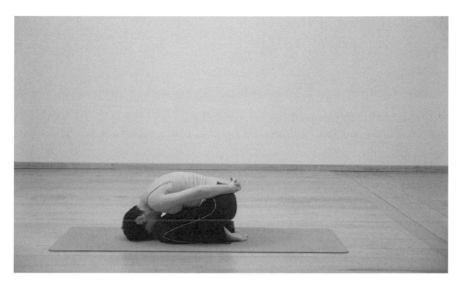

Figure 7.39. Great Gesture

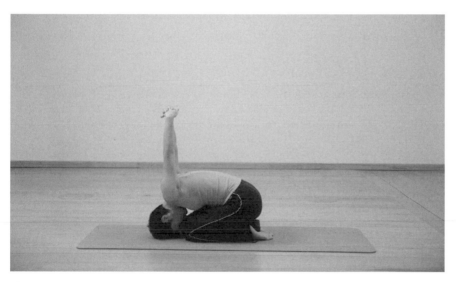

Figure 7.40. Great Gesture

● Finally, maintain the kneeling posture and feel the effects of the stretch and the strong exhalation and following inhalation. Close your eyes if you would like to.

Variation: You can do the great gesture in a standing or seated posture. Check under "Yoga exercises at work."

Alternate Nostril Breathing

Purpose: expands the breathing capacity, calms you, and helps you to concentrate.

Since alternate nostril breathing can be done almost everywhere, it should be a part of your yoga practice at home as well as at work. Check "Yoga at work" for details on this pranayama exercise.

Table Posture

Purpose: strengthens arm, leg, and belly muscles, flexes the back, and expands the breathing space.

- Come into the seated posture on the floor (see "basic stances for Yoga at home"). Bend both your legs and place your feet hip joint width apart on the ground. Place your hands behind your back, with fingers facing toward your back (Figure 7.41).
- Inhale and tighten your pelvis muscles while you are lifting your torso until your thighs, torso, neck, and head are on one level and parallel to the ground. Make sure your hands are underneath your shoulders and your ankles are underneath your knees (Figure 7.42).
- Exhale while you are moving back into the starting position.

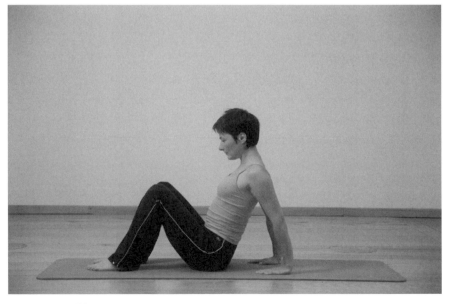

Figure 7.41. Table Posture

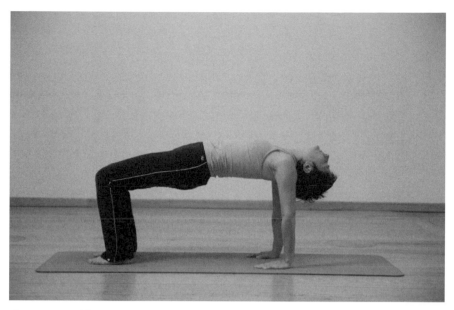

Figure 7.42. Table Posture

- Repeat the movement for six full inhalations and exhalations.
- Again come into the table posture and maintain it for three complete inhalations and exhalations.
- Finally, return to the seated posture and relax in a supine posture. Feel the space between your shoulder blades. Close your eyes, if it feels comfortable for you.

Fish Posture

Purpose: flexes the neck, shoulder and back, stretches the rip cage, and enlarges the upper breathing space.

- Come into the seated posture on the floor (see "supine posture" under basic stances for Yoga at home).
- Gently lower your torso backward and place your forearms on the ground. Make sure your elbows are underneath your shoulder joints (Figure 7.43).
- Inhale and bend your upper torso backward until the crown of your head touches the ground.
- Move your arms forward, and place your hands on top of your thighs near the groin. Lift your rip cage while your pelvis is kept on the ground (Figure 7.44).

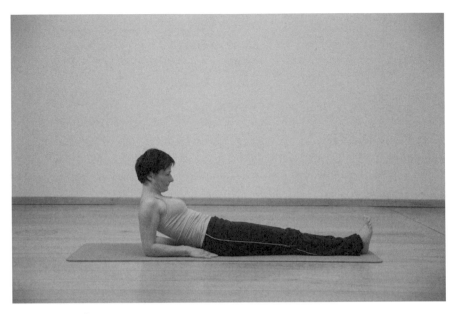

Figure 7.43. Fish Posture

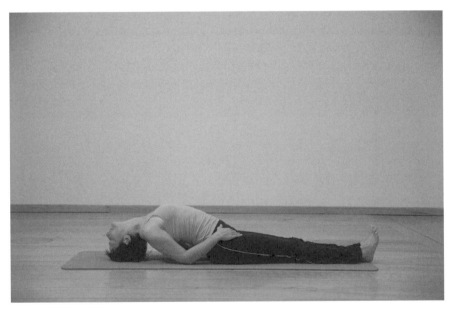

Figure 7.44. Fish Posture

- Maintain the position for six complete inhalations and exhalations.
- With an exhalation move your elbows and arms to the side and lower your torso.
- Feel the effects of the backward bend in your upper torso. Close your eyes if it feels comfortable.

Dynamic Asana

The sun salutation is a well-known series of yoga postures acknowledged by all schools and styles of yoga. In this series of asana, the flow of breathing and moving can easily be experienced. A proper sun salutation requires a lot of strength and flexibility. For our purposes, the sun salutation's little sister is more appropriate: the sunbird. It is a nicely flowing exercise during which the breathing is even and complete and is synchronized with the movements. The difference between body work and yoga can be seen in the breathing techniques.

At the same time the sunbird is a wonderful series of yoga asana that allow extensions into other postures: out of the tiger posture into the runner posture and out of the runner posture into the pyramid posture.

The sunbird is a combination of three core asana: the child, the tiger, and the mountain. In this series, you stretch and bend your shoulders and back and extend the stretch to your legs while doing the mountain. (Some yoga schools refer to the mountain as the downward facing dog. You may use whichever name you prefer.)

Contraindications

The sunbird is a very gentle way to stretch and bend and get into an inverted posture (mountain). However, it can be difficult for some people to kneel on their heels. Use a bolster (folded blanket) as a prop and put it under your knees or under your stretched feet.

People with uncontrolled high blood pressure and eye and ear conditions should keep their heads above heart level. They have to exercise with great caution and only do the easy mountain posture, which is described in Chapter 6, "Yoga Exercises at Work." This variation uses a chair or table for the mountain posture.

Alignment

Maintain the flow. Let the breathing guide your movements. Notice that the mountain posture is the ultimate posture with which to stretch the back as well as your arms and legs. A lot of people worry too much about the stretch of their legs. They forcefully lower their heels to the ground and bow their back. It is much better to stretch the back and bend the knees. After practicing for a while, the leg stretch will follow.

Core Asana: Sunbird

Child Posture

Purpose: arm and back stretch and strength.

- Come into the kneeling posture (see "basic stances for Yoga at home").
- Exhale while slowly bending your torso.
- Stretch out your arms and place your palms shoulder width apart on the floor. Make sure your fingers are straddled and your complete palms are lying on the ground (Figure 7.45).

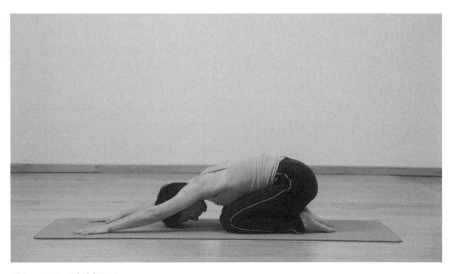

Figure 7.45. Child Posture

- Maintain the posture for six complete inhalations and exhalations.
- Slowly inhale while rolling up into the kneeling posture.
- Place your hands on your thighs and feel the effects with your eyes closed if you like.

Tiger Posture

Purpose: back bow and stretch.

- Come into the child posture (see the asana above).
- Inhale while you are rising into the tiger posture (kneeling on all fours). Make sure that your wrists are underneath your shoulders and your knees underneath your hip joints. These alignments help you to exercise without hurting your joints (Figure 7.46)
- Exhale while you are moving backward into the child position.
- Inhale and rise into the tiger position, exhale, and move backward into the child position.
- Repeat the movement for six complete inhalations and exhalations.
- To get back into the starting position, slowly inhale while rolling up into the kneeling position.
- Place your hands on your thighs and feel the effects with your eyes closed if you like.

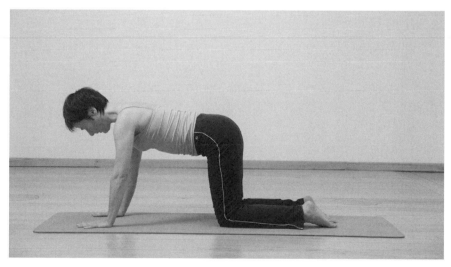

Figure 7.46. Tiger Posture

Mountain Posture

Purpose: arm, back, and leg stretch and strength.

- Come into the child posture (see the child posture asana).
- Inhale while you are rising into the tiger posture (kneeling on all fours). Make sure that your wrists are underneath your shoulders and your knees underneath your hip joints. Remember that your fingers are straddled and that your palms are completely pushing into the ground (this way the weight of your body is evenly distributed on both your hands). Tuck down your toes.
- Exhale, push your hands and toes into the ground, and lift your body upward. Make sure your arms and your back are completely stretched (Figure 7.47).
- Bend your knees if it helps to stretch your back.
- Maintain the position for six complete inhalations and exhalations.
- With an inhalation slowly walk with your feet toward your hands, bend your knees, and role up into the standing posture.
- Feel the stretch of your arms, back, and legs. Close your eyes, if it is comfortable for you.

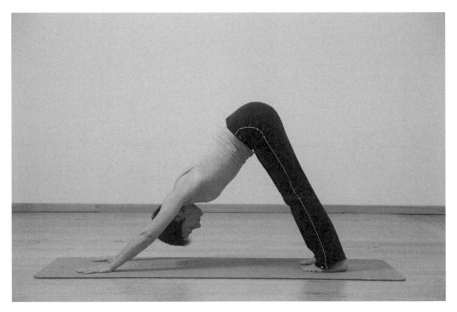

Figure 7.47. Mountain Posture

Variation 1: If you cannot easily place your heels on the ground while practicing the mountain posture, keep your knees bent and do alternating stretches of the legs. Stretch one leg and bring the heel to the ground. Then do the other leg.

Variation 2: To feel the stretch in your arms, back, legs, and in your flanks, you have to extend the movement of the alternating stretches of the legs to alternating twists of your pelvis. Bend one leg, slightly move it inward, and twist the same side of your pelvis. You can feel the stretch starting underneath your arm, over the pelvis, down your leg, and in your heel.

Variation 3: If you suffer from glaucoma, a detached retina, ear inflammation, or uncontrolled high blood pressure, keep your head above heart level. Use the back of a chair as a prop (check easy mountain in Chapter 6, "Yoga Exercises at Work").

Sunbird: The Combination of Child Posture, Tiger Posture, and Mountain Posture

- Come into the child posture.
- Inhale while you are rising into the tiger posture (kneeling on all fours). Make sure that your wrists are underneath your shoulders and your knees underneath your hip joints. Remember that your fingers are straddled and that your palms are completely pushing into the ground. Tuck down your toes.
- Exhale, push your hands and toes into the ground, and lift your body upward into the mountain posture. Make sure your arms and your back are completely stretched. Bend your knees if it helps to stretch your back.
- Inhale while lowering your body back into the tiger posture.
- Exhale while moving backward into the child posture.
- Inhale while rising into the tiger posture.
- Exhale while rising into the mountain posture.
- Inhale while lowering your body back into the tiger posture.
- Exhale while moving backward into the child posture.
- Repeat the combination in your breathing rhythm.
- Finally, return to the kneeling posture and feel the effect of the sunbird asana.

Variation: Add the folded leaf posture to take a break. The folded leaf posture follows the child posture. You can either place your hands at the side of your body resting your head on the mat or you can place your hands in front of you (one hand on top of the other) resting your head on your upper hand.

Elective Asana

Threading the Needle

Purpose: enhances the flexibility of the shoulders and stretches the muscles of the upper torso.

- Come into the tiger posture (see tiger posture asana). Make sure that your wrists are underneath your shoulders and that your knees are underneath your hip joints. These alignments help you to exercise without hurting your joints (Figure 7.48).
- Exhale while you are moving your right hand sideway underneath your left arm and shoulder. The palm is facing upward (Figure 7.49).
- Inhale while moving back into the starting position.

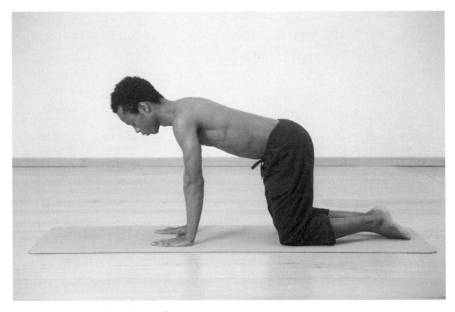

Figure 7.48. Threading the Needle

- Do the movement on both sides during six complete exhalations and inhalations.
- With the next exhalation keep the position, rest your head on one side, and stretch out your upper arm. Maintain the asana for three complete inhalations and exhalations (Figure 7.50).

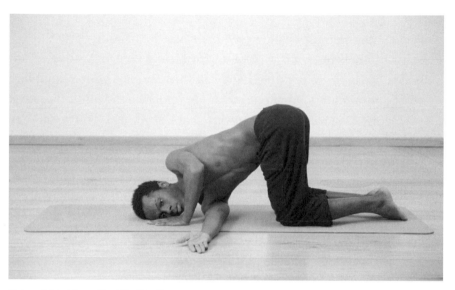

Figure 7.49. *Threading the Needle*

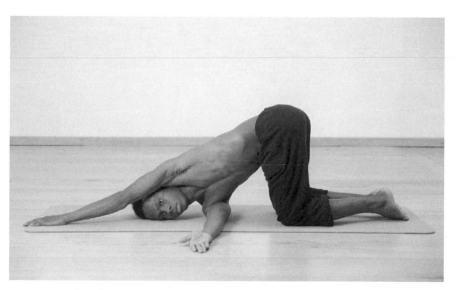

Figure 7.50. *Threading the Needle*

- Inhale and return to the starting position.
- Exhale again and do the asana on the other side.
- Finally, return to the kneeling posture and place your fingers on top of your thighs. Feel the effects with your eyes closed if you like.

Runner Posture

Purpose: legs and spine stretch and strength.

- Come into the tiger posture (see tiger posture asana).
- Inhale and bring your right foot forward. Place it between your hands. Stretch your other leg backward. Check your alignment: wrist underneath your shoulder, ankle underneath your knee, neck is stretched, face looking downward, back stretched, pelvis muscles tight, leg stretched, and the heel pushing backward toward the floor (Figure 7.51).
- Maintain the position for six full inhalations and exhalations.
- Exhale while pushing up your body and placing the front foot next to the other: the mountain posture.
- Inhale and move into the tiger posture.
- Exhale and move into the child posture.
- Finally, you can either rest in the folded leaf posture or roll up into the kneeling posture.
- Feel the effect of the whole exercise.

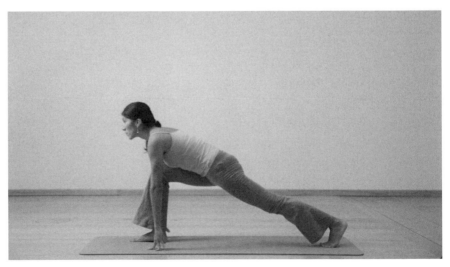

Figure 7.51. Runner Posture

Variations: If you have strong legs, strong back muscles, and good balance, take your hands off the mat while you are in the runner posture. Stretch out your arms without pulling up your shoulders and bend backward (Figure 7.52). The posture is less challenging if you place the knee of your back leg on the floor (Figure 7.53).

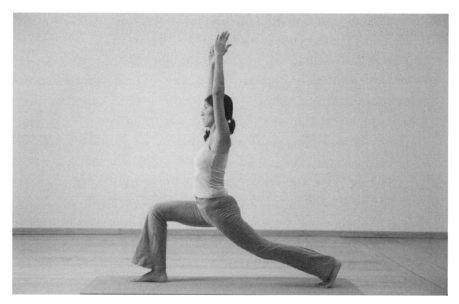

Figure 7.52. Runner Posture

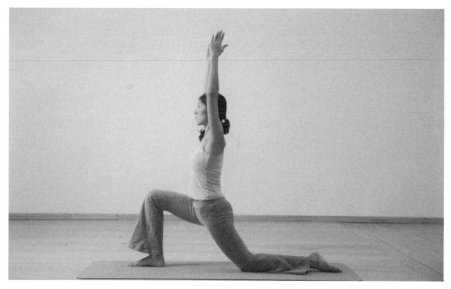

Figure 7.53. Runner Posture

Pyramid Posture

Purpose: legs and spine stretch.

- Come into the standing posture (see "basic stances for Yoga at work").
- Bring your feet one leg length apart. Make sure both soles and both outer sides of your feet are touching the ground. Bend your knees.
- Inhale and stretch out your spine.
- Exhale while slowly bending down your torso until the tips of your fingers touch the floor. Stretch your knees. Your wrists are underneath your shoulders. Always maintain this position (Figure 7.54).
- With the next exhalation slowly bend your right knee. Make sure that both outer sides of your feet are still on the floor (Figure 7.55).
- Inhale while slowly moving back into the starting position.
- Exhale while slowly bending your left knee (Figure 7.56).
- Inhale while slowly moving back into the starting position.
- Repeat the bends and stretches for six complete inhalations and exhalations.
- Bend your knees, inhale, and slowly roll your torso upward.
- Bring your feet closer together and come into the standing posture. Feel the effects of the exercise. Close your eyes if you like.

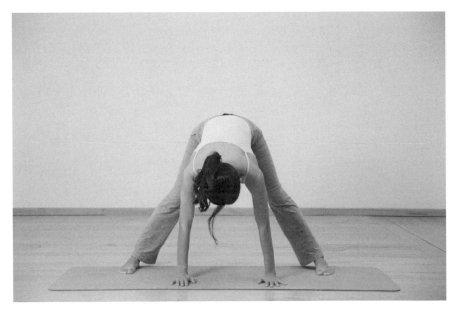

Figure 7.54. Pyramid Posture

Variation: If your back is rounded while your fingertips are on the floor, put a thick book (two books) or a little stool in front of you.

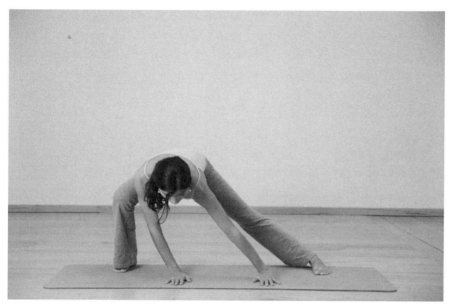

Figure 7.55. Pyramid Posture

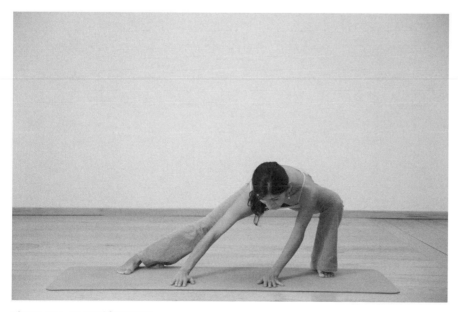

Figure 7.56. Pyramid Posture

Triangle Posture

Purpose: stretches the flanks.

- Come into the standing posture (see "basic stances for Yoga at work"). Turn your right foot outward with the toes pointing forward. Turn the left foot 45 degrees inward.
- Inhale while raising your arms over the sides until they are fully stretched out at shoulder height (Figure 7.57). Make sure that you do not pull up your shoulders. If you are not exactly sure, raise your shoulders briefly and let them sink again.
- Exhale while bending your torso to the right side. Both arms are stretched (Figure 7.58). Continue the movement pointing your right arm downward and your left arm upward. Make sure you do not bend your torso forward. Keep both your flanks stretched. Keep your head and neck straight (Figure 7.59).
- Maintain the posture for six complete inhalations and exhalations.
- With an inhalation return to the upright position and place both your feet closer together. Compare both sides of your body: your legs, both sides of your pelvis, both sides of your shoulders, and your face.

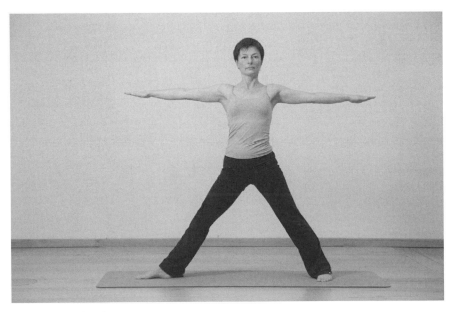

Figure 7.57. Triangle Posture

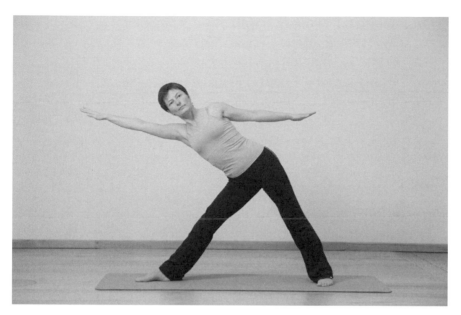

Figure 7.58. Triangle Posture

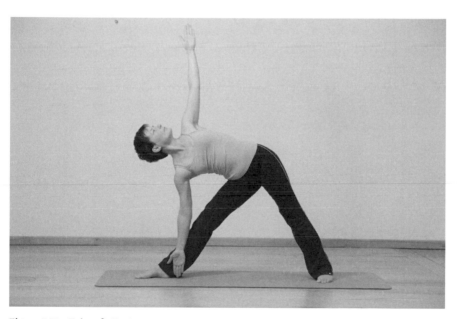

Figure 7.59. Triangle Posture

- Turn your left foot outward with the toes pointing forward. Turn the right foot 45 degrees inward.
- Exhale and bend to the other side.
- Maintain the posture for six complete inhalations and exhalations.
- Finally, with an inhalation return to the upright position and place both your feet closer together. Feel the effects of the stretches in your flanks. Close your eyes if it is pleasant for you to do so.

Boat Posture

Purpose: abdominal strength.

- Come into the seated posture on the floor (see "basic stances").
- Place your hands behind your back, fingers facing toward the back. The pelvis is upright, the entire length of your spinal column is stretched, your head crown extends upward, and your sternum is raised.
- Bend your knees and position your feet flat on the floor hip joint width apart from one another. Your face and mouth are relaxed. Breathe completely in and out through your nose.
- While you inhale stretch and lift your legs with your feet bent (Figure 7.60).
- Maintain the posture during six complete inhalations and exhalations.

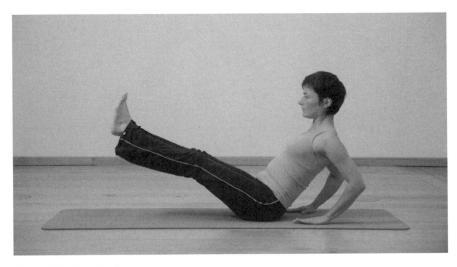

Figure 7.60. Boat Posture

● Get back into the seated posture with an exhalation and feel the effects. Close your eyes if it is pleasant for you.

Variation 1: If you do not have the strength to keep the posture, exercise in a more relaxed way and keep one leg on the ground (Figure 7.61).

Variation 2: If you want to do the exercise more vigorously, do the exercise without using your arms and hands as a support (Figure 7.62).

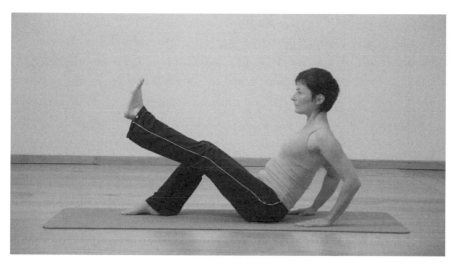

Figure 7.61. Boat Posture

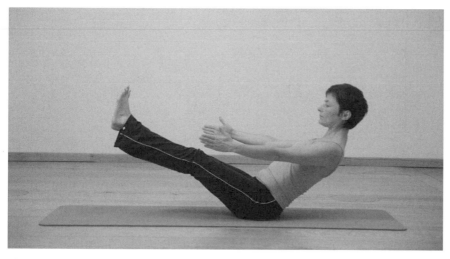

Figure 7.62. Boat Posture

Cow Posture

Purpose: stretches neck, shoulders, and arms.

- Come into the seated posture on the floor (see "basic stances"). Bend your left leg and place your left foot at the outer side of your right hip. Bend your right leg and place your right foot at the outer side of your left hip. Make sure both knees are in line and your weight is evenly distributed on both your sit bones (make sure that you do not tilt to one side) (Figure 7.63).
- Inhale while you are lifting your left arm.
- Exhale and bend your left arm.
- Inhale while you are moving your right arm behind your torso.
- Exhale and bend your right arm until both your hands meet.
- Turn your head and look upward to your left elbow (Figure 7.64).
- Maintain the posture for six complete inhalations and exhalations.
- With an exhalation lower both arms and place them on your thighs. Compare the feeling in both sides of your body: both sides of your face, both your arms, and your shoulders.
- Change the position of your legs and repeat the posture to the other side with your left knee on top and your right elbow raised (Figure 7.65).

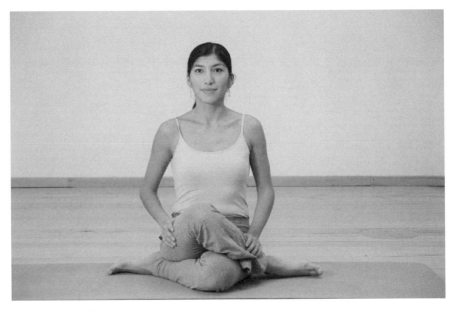

Figure 7.63. Cow Posture

● Finally, come into the seated posture and feel the effect of the whole asana. Close your eyes if you like.

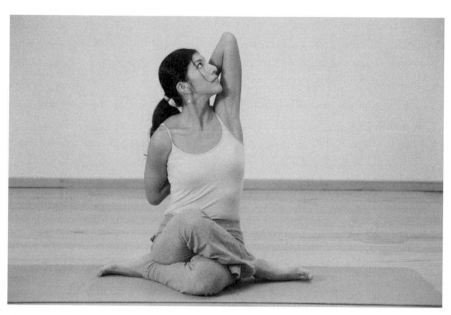

Figure 7.64. Cow Posture

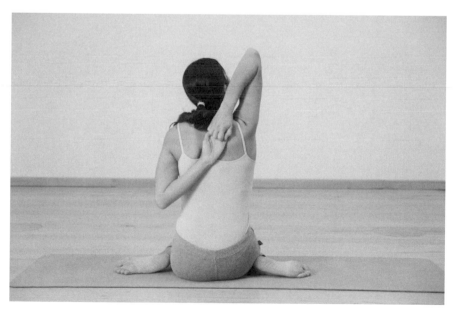

Figure 7.65. Cow Posture

Realign Again

Shoulder Bridge

Purpose: flexibility and strength of the back and leg muscles.

- Come into the supine posture on the floor (see "basic stances").
- Bend both your legs and place your feet hip joint width apart on the mat.
- Place your arms on the mat next to your sides. Your palms are facing downward (Figure 7.66).
- Inhale through your nose and tighten your bottom or rather your pelvis muscles while lifting your back vertebrae by vertebrae (Figure 7.67).
- Exhale through your nose while lowering your back vertebrae by vertebrae. Relax your pelvis muscles at the end of the movement.
- Make sure your breathing and moving are completely synchronized.
- Repeat the movements for six complete inhalations and exhalations.
- To do the complete asana, inhale through your nose and tighten your bottom—or rather your pelvis muscles—while lifting your back vertebrae by vertebrae. Make sure your soles push into the mat.
- Bring your arms closer together and remain on the outer side of your arms. Close your hands under your bending back (Figure 7.68).

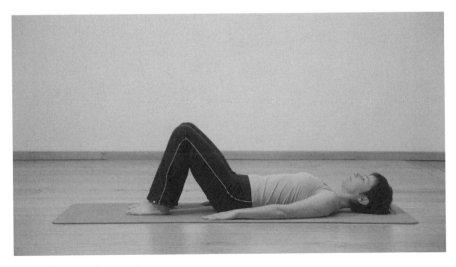

Figure 7.66. Shoulder Bridge

- Maintain the posture for six complete inhalations and exhalations. Get as much space between your upper spine and the mat as possible without hurting yourself.
- To get out of the posture, place your arms and hands at the side of your body and exhale while you are lowering your spine vertebrae by vertebrae. Relax your pelvic muscles.
- Stretch out your legs and feel the effects of the back bow. Close your eyes if it feels comfortable.

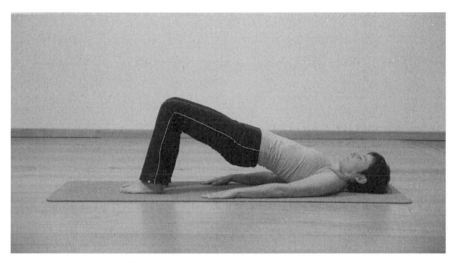

Figure 7.67. Shoulder Bridge

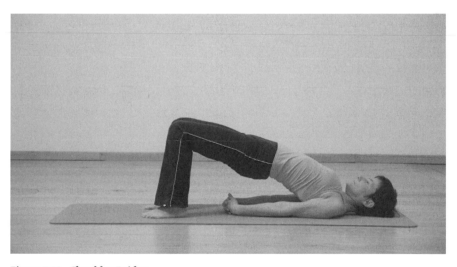

Figure 7.68. Shoulder Bridge

Crocodile Posture

Purpose: flexibility and strength of the belly muscles.

- Lie on your back (supine posture), bend both your knees, and place both your feet hip joint width apart on the ground.
- Stretch out your arms at shoulder level. Completely relax your shoulders and keep them on the ground. The palms are facing downward.
- Slowly lift your knees toward your chest. Make sure that your neck is stretched and that both your lower legs and feet are relaxed (Figure 7.69).
- Exhale through your nose while you are moving your knees to the left side and your head to the right side. Start with small movements (Figure 7.70).
- Inhale through your nose while you are moving your head and knees back into the middle.
- Repeat the movement for six complete inhalations and exhalations. Extend the movement with each exhalation.
- To maintain the position and do the asana, place your feet back on the mat. Place your pelvis further to the right until your weight is

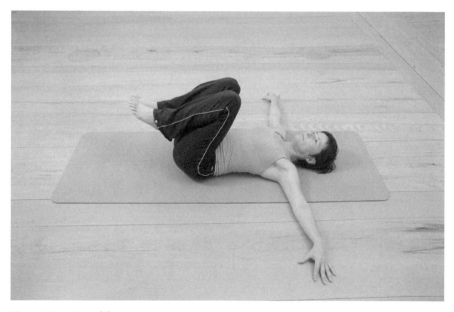

Figure 7.69. Crocodile Posture

on the left side of your bottom. Bend your knees again and lift them toward your chest.

- Exhale while moving the knees completely to the left side and your head to the right side. Make sure that both shoulders are still on the mat and that your neck is still stretched. Rest your left hand on your right knee (Figure 7.71).

- Maintain the posture for six complete inhalations and exhalations. You may close your eyes if you like. The more you relax, the easier it is to stay in this posture.

- With an inhalation turn back into the starting position and compare the feeling in both sides of your body: both legs, both sides of the pelvis, both sides of your shoulders, and your face.

- Repeat the asana to the other side.

- Finally, stretch out on your back and feel the effect of the complete asana.

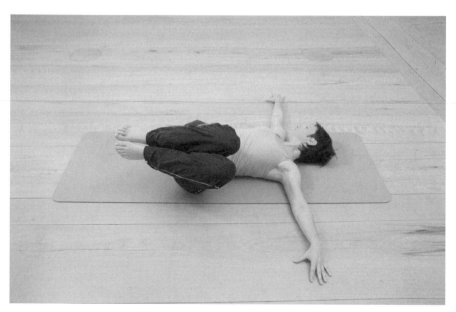

Figure 7.70. Crocodile Posture

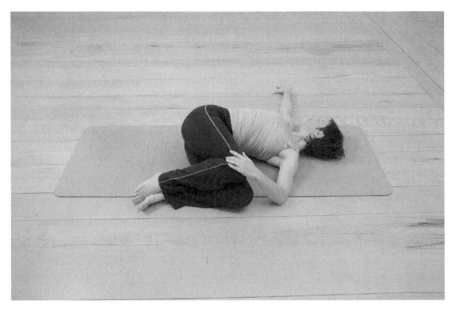

Figure 7.71. Crocodile Posture

Relax and Become Aware of the Effects

At the end of the yoga class, it is important to bring in the harvest. After all the stretching and strengthening, the dynamic and aligning postures, and the breathing exercises, you should give yourself a little time to relax and become aware of the effects of the asana.

To enable you to compare your physical and mental being before and after the yoga class, it is useful to always begin and end with one classic asana. I propose that you use the shanti asana.

At the end of the relaxing posture, you should get into a seated posture to stabilize your blood circulation. Depending on your personal preferences and abilities, you can choose from the four seated postures.

Core Asana

Shanti Asana

Purpose: complete relaxation and deepening of the effects.

Each posture is described in detail at the beginning of this chapter.

Free Seat

Purpose: a gentle stretch for the hips that stabilizes blood circulation and provides a moment to feel the effects of yoga.

Elective Asana

Kneeling Posture

Purpose: provides an elevated posture to stabilize the blood circulation and feel the effects of the program on body and mind.

Half Lotus or Complete Lotus Seat

Purpose: stable posture to become aware of the effects yoga offers by profoundly stretching the pelvis and legs.

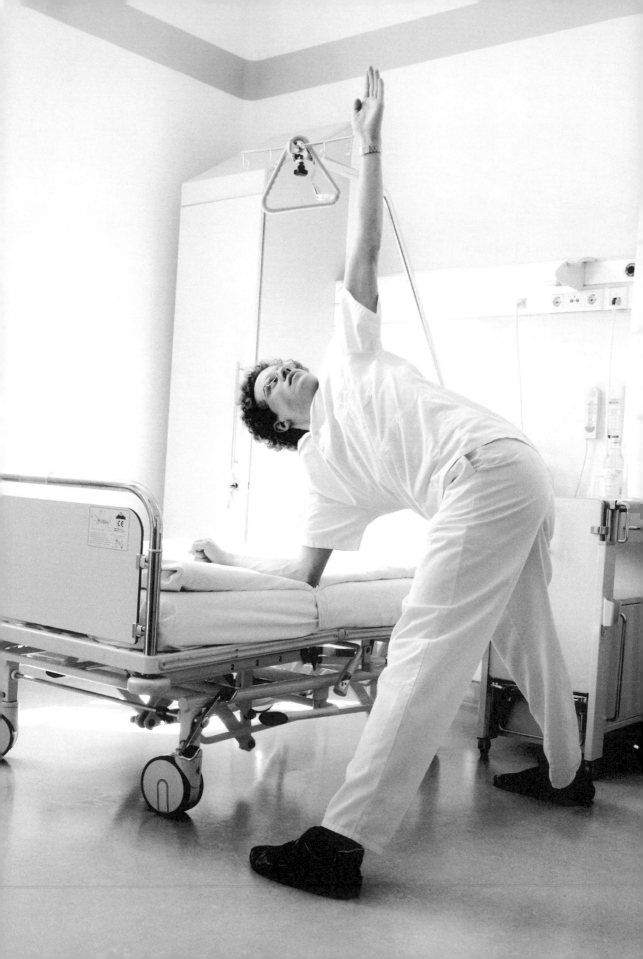

Advanced Yoga Practice

8

As an advanced yoga practitioner, you may be interested in reading and learning more about the asana. With the help of the following discussion of advanced asana, you can individually deepen and broaden your yoga practice and knowledge.

These asana can provide answers to your individual needs, such as a special stretch or a new practice to enable you to relax, so you can complement your yoga program with these asana. During a 90 minute program of yoga, these advanced asana should follow the sun bird asana.

The asana are presented in groups following the classic distinction of forward, backward, and sideward bends, inversions, twists, and balancing postures. In addition, there is additional information on the eye exercises that were already described in Chapter 6.

For each group of asana the definition, the proper alignment and the contraindications are given. With the help of the detailed explanation of two asana per group, you can learn and practice the proper performance and experience the effects. This way you learn to practice yoga with consciousness and become able to use all variations of an asana depending on your actual fitness level, which varies from day to day.

Advanced Asana

Forward Bends	Head to Knee Posture
	Turtle Posture
Backward Bends	Standing Bow Posture
	Lying Bow Posture
Sideward Bends	Half-Moon Posture
	Side Angle Posture
Inversions	Half Shoulderstand
	Full Shoulderstand

Twists	Torso Rotation
	Twisted Triangle Posture
Balancing Postures	Hero 3 Posture
	Eagle Posture
Eye Exercises	Lying Eight
	Near and Distant View
	Cupping and Blinking

Forward Bends

All exercises in which the back or dorsal side of the spinal column is stretched and the front or ventral side is bent are called forward bends. Most often these bends follow a standing posture or a seated posture. Forward bends can also occur when you are on your back and are moving your legs toward your stomach. In this position, you can feel your lower spine lifting upward and away from the mat or floor.

Their Purposes

All forward bends stretch the muscles of the back of your legs, your pelvis, and your back. They also stretch the joint between the pelvis and spine. Underdeveloped muscles in the back, as well as of the belly, are the cause of poor pelvis alignment. The pelvis is tilted forward, with the spine bent slightly forward in its lower part and often rounded in its upper part. This poor posture is a serious problem. Yoga helps you to detect this position and keep you upright without feeling unnatural. Exercising forward bends develops your flexibility, gives you a feeling of energy, and enables you to completely inhale and exhale.

Forward bends are very common movements in daily life. They are the most used positions for people working as health professionals. Examples include standing in the operating room leaning forward over

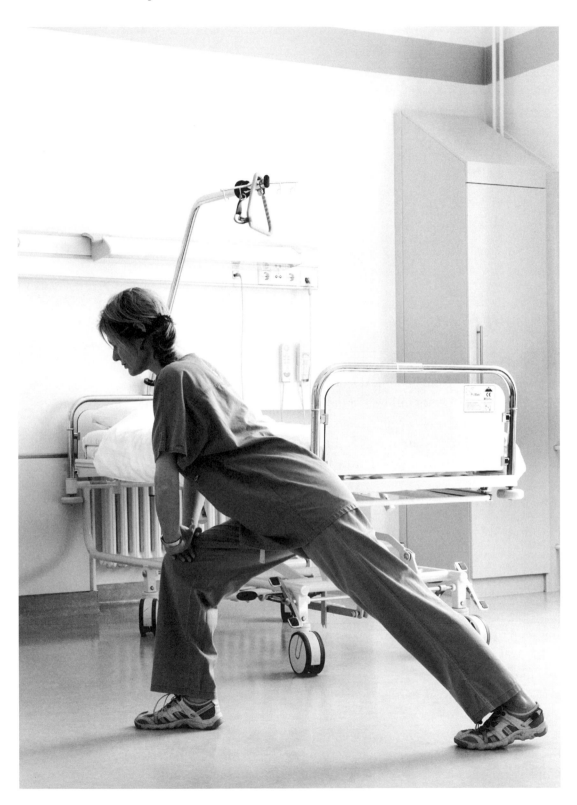

the patient, on the ward serving food to a patient, and in the laboratory working at the table. As long as your back does not trouble you, you might not even notice that you are in this position. But if you have problems with your back, you might feel a flare when you are stretching to get into an upright position. These painful movements often follow unconscious forward bends that are accompanied by heavy lifting—especially if you do the lifting completely using your back muscles (knees are stretched and the back is rounded). A sudden movement or heavy lifting may cause sudden pain that immediately stops you. You feel unable to stretch and stand up.

Contraindication

Forward bends should not be practiced if you feel acute pain in your back or stomach. People with uncontrolled high blood pressure or eye and ear conditions should not lower their heads below their heart level.

Alignment

While practicing forward bends, many yoga students focus on the wrong concern: Can I touch the ground, and does my front touch my knees? They forget about the most important part of the exercise: Is my spine fully stretched out? A forward bend without stretching the vertebrae is a cause of backaches in everyday life, as well as when doing yoga.

Head to Knee Posture

- Take a seat on the floor and distribute your weight evenly over both sit bones. Position your feet hip joint width apart from one another and bend your feet (pull your toes and feet in the direction of your torso). Make sure that your pelvis is in an upright position. To check your pose, place your hand behind your back and stretch. Maintain the position and relax your arms on your thighs.
- Inhale while you are lifting your arms and stretching your spinal column along its entire length (Figure 8.1).
- Exhale while bending your torso forward. Make sure that your spine is always stretched, including the neck. Do not bow your head backward (Figure 8.2).
- Inhale while stretching your torso again in the forward bend.
- Exhale and bend forward again.

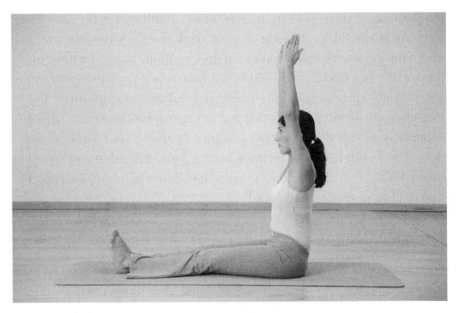

Figure 8.1. Head to Knee Posture

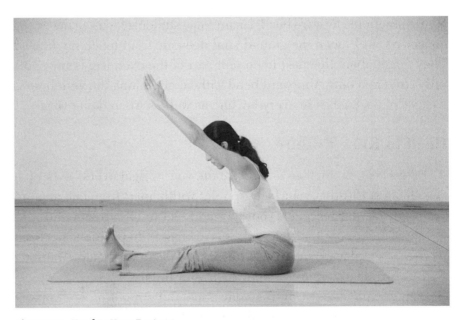

Figure 8.2. Head to Knee Posture

- Maintain the position for six complete inhalations and exhalations.
- Inhale again and rise into an upright posture. Feel the effects of the stretch in the back of your legs, in your pelvis, and in your back.
- As a counterstretch, come into the squat position, embrace your knees with your arms, bend your head forward, and relax your back.

Turtle Posture

- Take a seat on the floor and distribute your weight evenly over both sit bones. Bend your knees and bring your soles together. Make sure that your pelvis is in an upright position. To check your pose, place your hand behind your back and stretch. Maintain the position and relax your hands on your ankles (Figure 8.3).
- Inhale through your nose while stretching your spine.
- Exhale through your nose while bending your torso forward from your hip joints. Place your forearms on your mat and rest for an inhalation (Figure 8.4).
- Maintain the posture for six complete inhalations and exhalations.
- To release the position inhale while slowly rolling up your body and return to the seated posture.
- Feel the effects of the strong forward bend for a moment and, if it is comfortable for you, close your eyes.

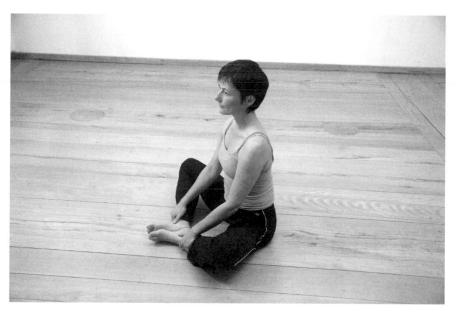

Figure 8.3. Turtle Posture

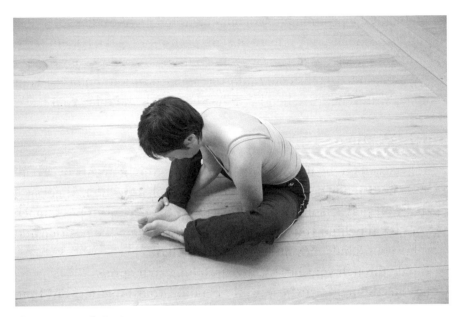

Figure 8.4. *Turtle Posture*

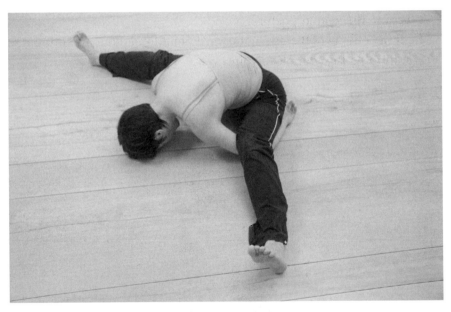

Figure 8.5. *Turtle Posture*

● As a counterstretch, do some rounds of the crocodile posture (see Figure 7.10).

Variation 1: If you feel like stretching even more, come into the above detailed posture and stretch your legs to the side. With an exhalation, let your arms and hands further slide backward underneath your thighs. Relax your head and drop your shoulders. Breathe completely and evenly in and out through your nose and hold this position for six complete inhalations and exhalations. Close your eyes if it feels comfortable (Figure 8.5).

Variation 2: If you need to develop flexibility to get into the turtle posture, start with the variation on a chair (see Chapter 6, "Yoga Exercises at Work").

Backward Bends

In backward bends the front or ventral side of the body is stretched and the back or dorsal side is bent. Backward bends follow a standing posture mostly with raised and stretched arms, that is, the standing bow posture or opening of the sun salutation. Backward bends can also be done when lying on the stomach and lifting the upper torso as in the cobra or sphinx posture or with a leg lift as in the lying bow posture.

All backward bends increase the strength of the back muscles, straighten the pelvis, and expand the muscles of the chest and entire front of the body.

The breathing space opens and allows complete inhalations and exhalations. A feeling of energy and power ensues.

Their Purposes

Back bends enhance the flexibility of the upper back. While the upper back is mostly bent forward, a hump back is often noticeable. People working long hours in front of computers often show this round shape of their upper back.

People who tend to always rush and do a lot of things at the same time tend to bow forward. A side view shows that their upper body is not in line with their pelvis and legs. It is good for them to slowly bend

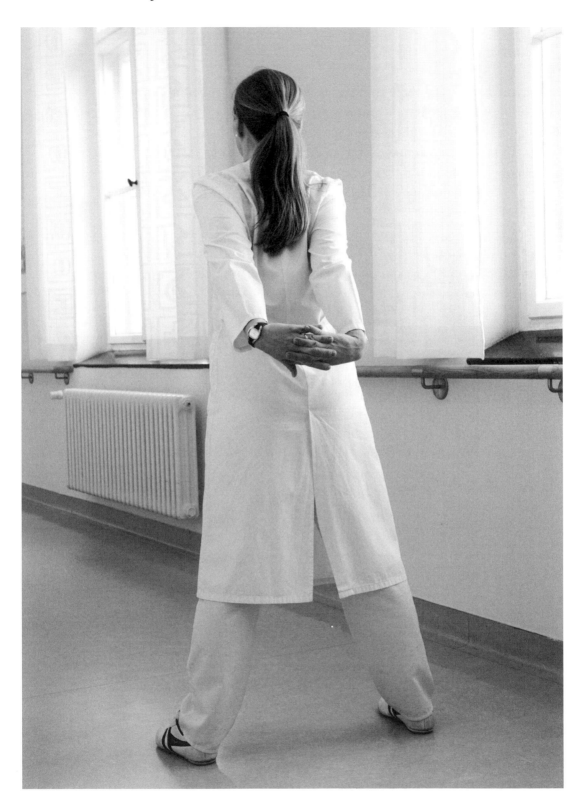

their upper torso backward and to realign it. For them, the conscious exercise of a back bend is also helpful mentally: The slow practice of backward bends helps them to concentrate, to stay in line, and to be focused.

Contraindication

Many people suffer from back problems as a result of poor posture and weak muscles. If their soreness is in the upper spine, they often have a stiff neck or cannot fully move their heads. If the problem is located in the lower back, they feel sudden pain and sometimes are unable to move. Though back bends are very good to build muscles and improve flexibility, they have to be introduced very slowly. The first step is to fully stretch out the spinal column and tighten the pelvis muscles.

Alignment

Two things are most important when performing the back stretch: (1) the pelvis muscles have to be tightened to guarantee an upright position and (2) the spinal column has to be fully stretched out. For someone with back problems, it is more useful to think of lengthening the spinal column than bending it backward.

Standing Bow Posture

- Come into the standing posture and tighten your pelvis muscles. Shift your weight to the right foot and leg. Bend your left knee, move both arms backward, and hold your left foot with both your hands (Figure 8.6).
- Inhale through your nose while stretching your spine again in this position.
- Exhale through your nose while slowly bending your left thigh backward.
- With the next inhalation stretch your spine again in this position.
- With the following exhalation slowly bend your left thigh further backward. Make sure that your left leg is not rotating to the side (Figure 8.7).
- If you feel the impulse to extend the bow, slowly bend backward and hold the posture again. Maintain the posture for six complete inhalations and exhalations.

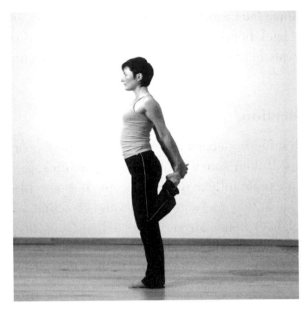

Figure 8.6. Standing Bow Posture

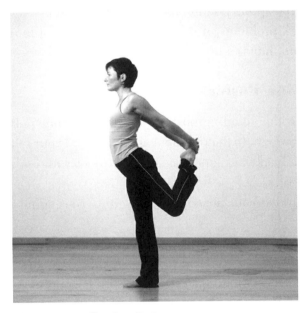

Figure 8.7. Standing Bow Posture

- To get out of the posture, slowly release the foot and bring your thigh forward with an inhalation. Take hold of your knee. Exhale and pull your knee close to your chest. Inhale and stretch your spine again in this position.
- With an exhalation, release your knee, stretch your leg, and place your left foot on the ground.
- Compare both sides of your body: your legs, both sides of your pelvis, your shoulders, and both sides of your face.
- Repeat the posture on the other side.
- Finally, get back into the starting position. Feel the effects of the back bend in the standing posture. Close your eyes if it is pleasant for you.
- As a counterstretch, bend your knees. Exhale while bending your stretched torso forward. Relax your neck. Place your elbows on your knees or cross your arms and let them hang down.

Lying Bow Posture

- Lie on your back. Inhale and stretch out your left arm. Exhale and slowly turn to the left until you lie on your stomach.
- When you are on your stomach, place your arms at your sides with the palms facing downward.
- Tighten your pelvis muscles and keep them tight during the whole asana.
- Bend both your knees and move your hands closer together behind your back until you can grip your ankles. Stretch your spine again in this position and make sure that you do not bend your head backward. Keep your front on the mat (Figure 8.8).
- With the next inhalation lift your torso and your thighs. To extend the back bend, inhale and further bend backward. Maintain the position for six complete inhalations and exhalations (Figure 8.9).
- To get out of the posture lower your legs and arms with an exhalation. Turn your head to the side and rest your head on one ear. Place your arms at your sides with your palms facing upward. Let both heels glide to the sides.
- Feel the effects of this posture. Close your eyes if it feels good to you.
- Stretch your right arm and turn right until you lie on your back again.
- As a counterstretch, do some rounds of the knee to the chest posture (see Figures 7.11 and 7.12).

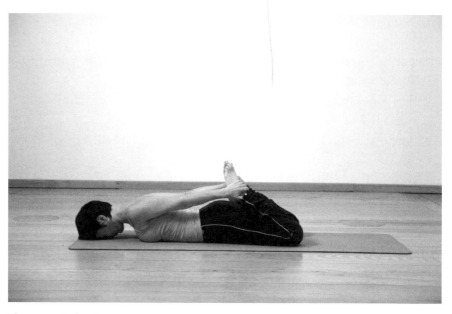

Figure 8.8. Lying Bow Posture

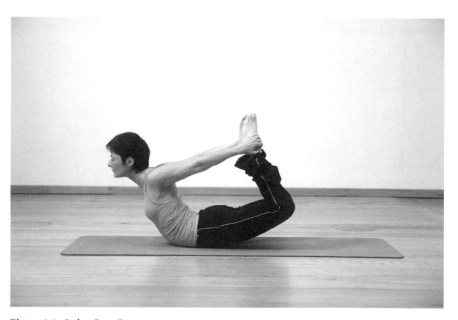

Figure 8.9. Lying Bow Posture

Sideward Bends

Bends of the spine toward one side are rare in everyday life. They are most often combined with forward bends. Yoga helps to focus attention on this unusual direction of movement and makes it possible to differentiate between forward and sideward bends. A feeling of greater flexibility goes along with a profound stretch of the flanks. If the stretch is done to one side the polarity of the body can unmistakably be experienced. To counterbalance weaknesses the exercises can be done more often or more vigorously on the weaker side.

Their Purposes

While bending to the side, the muscles of the flanks and between the rips get stretched. The stretch can be enhanced if the shoulders and arms are involved in the movement. The power and flexibility of the flank muscles define the stability of the pelvis and enable the upright stretch of the lumbar vertebrae or lower back. Unbalanced working positions or the tendency to tilt the head and shoulders to one side lead to a crooked spinal column. Sideward bends are counterstretches for these poor postures.

Contraindication

People with acute back pain should start their practice with stretches and small side bends. If you have a stiff neck that hurts apply warmth: Stretch out on a warm blanket and use an electric pad or hot water bottle. Threading the needle (see Figures 7.48, 7.49, and 7.50) is one of the best yoga postures to prevent further suffering from a stiff neck or tension in the upper back, shoulders, and neck. Warmth is also good if you have pain in your lower back. Start with small side bends (see Figure 7.10) and do some rotations of your pelvis (hula hoop style) while you are standing upright and resting your hands on your pelvis.

Alignment

To get the desired results, side bends have to be done with a stretched spine and strictly to the side. Flanks and rips do not benefit you if you bow to the side while bending forward. Do not worry about the extension. Be sure you stretch the flanks and stay in a side bend.

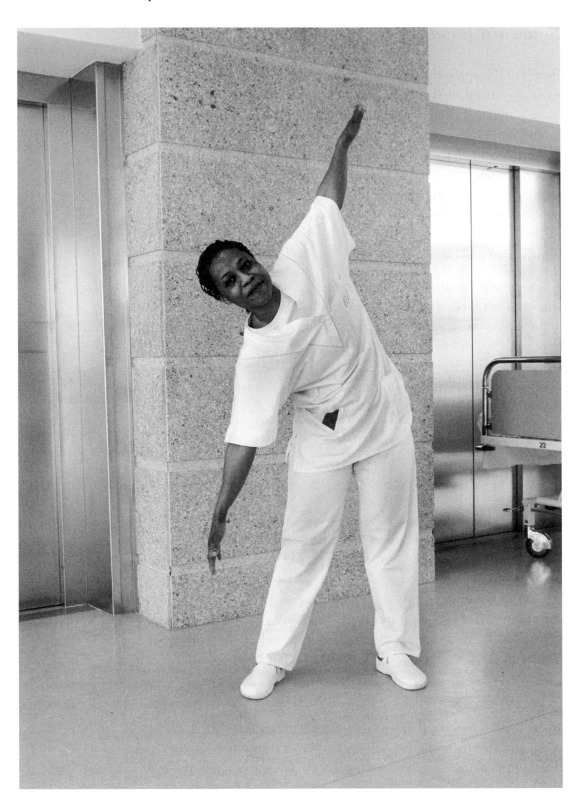

Half Moon Posture

- Come into the standing posture and position your feet one length of a leg apart. Turn the right foot outward with the toes pointing forward. Turn the left foot approximately 45 degrees inward.
- Breathe in through your nose while slowly lifting your arms over your sides until they are fully stretched out at shoulder height (Figure 8.10). Make sure that you do not pull up your shoulders. If you are not exactly sure, raise your shoulders briefly and let them sink again.
- Exhale and bend your right knee and place the fingertips of your right hand in front of your right foot to the right. Your left arm is relaxed and your left hand is on top of your pelvis (Figure 8.11).
- Inhale and stretch your right leg and lift your left leg and left arm. In the proper alignment the left leg is parallel to the floor and the left arm is in line with the right arm. Your neck is stretched and your head in a balanced position looking forward (Figure 8.12).
- Maintain the posture for six complete inhalations and exhalations.
- To get out of the posture inhale and push your right hand against the floor and lift your torso and right arm while lowering your left leg and arm.

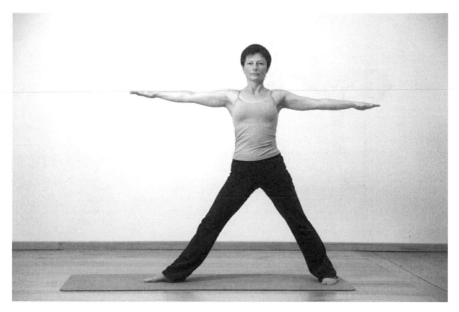

Figure 8.10. Half-Moon Posture

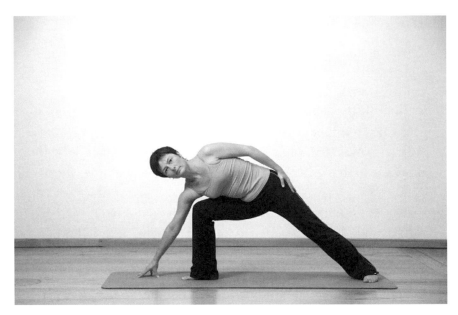

Figure 8.11. Half-Moon Posture

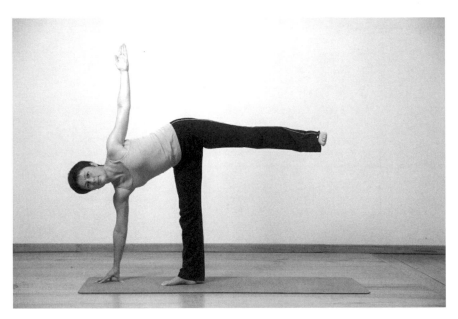

Figure 8.12. Half-Moon Posture

- Come into the standing posture and compare the feeling in both sides of your body: your legs, both sides of your pelvis, both shoulders, and both sides of your face. You may close your eyes if you like.
- Repeat the posture on the other side.
- Finally, take up the standing posture, compare both sides again, and feel the effects of the whole balancing exercise. Close your eyes if it is pleasant for you.
- As a counterstretch, do a torso rotation (see Figures 6.23 and 6.24).

Variation: If it is difficult for you to get into or keep the posture, you can practice in front of a wall and stay in touch with it during the whole exercise. In the beginning, it is a very good pose to help you getting properly aligned.

Side Angle Posture

- Come into the standing posture. Position your feet one length of a leg apart. Turn the right foot outward with the toes pointing forward. Turn the left foot approximately 45 degrees inward.
- Inhale while slowly raising your arms over your sides until they are fully stretched and at shoulder height. Make sure that you do not pull up your shoulders. If you are not exactly sure, raise your shoulders briefly and let them sink again.
- Exhale while bending your right knee and moving your torso and arms to the right (Figure 8.13).
- Inhale and rest in this position.
- Exhale while bending your right arm and placing your right forearm on your right thigh. Your left arm is stretched and your palm is facing the right side. Make sure you do not bend forward (Figure 8.14).
- Inhale and rest in this position.
- With the next exhalation stretch your right arm and lower your right hand in front of your bent knee until you can place your fingertips or your hand on the ground. Make sure you are not bending forward (Figure 8.15). Your head is turned upward looking toward the ceiling.
- Maintain the posture for six complete inhalations and exhalations.
- Inhale and move out of the posture lifting your torso and lowering your arms.

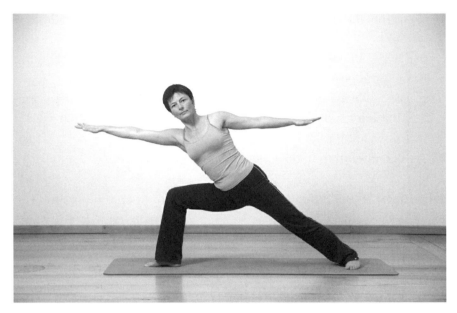

Figure 8.13. Side Angle Posture

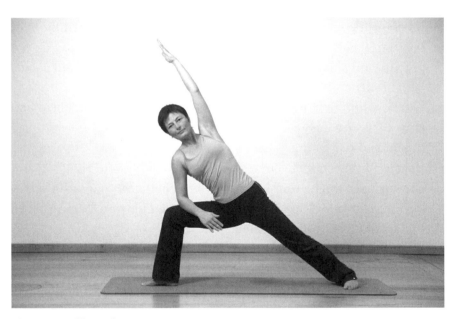

Figure 8.14. Side Angle Posture

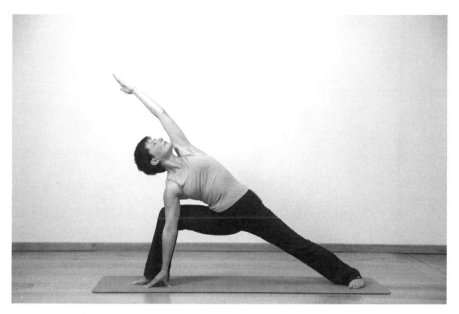

Figure 8.15. Side Angle Posture

- Compare both sides of your body in the starting position. Feel both legs, both sides of your pelvis, your shoulders, and both sides of your face.
- Repeat the exercise on the other side.
- Finally, get into the standing posture and feel the effects of the whole exercise. Close your eyes if it is pleasant for you.
- As a counterstretch, bend your knees. Exhale while bending your stretched torso forward. Relax your neck. Place your elbows on your knees or cross your arms and let them hang down.

Variation: If you have problems with the head pose (looking upward while bending to the side), keep your head in a balanced posture facing forward.

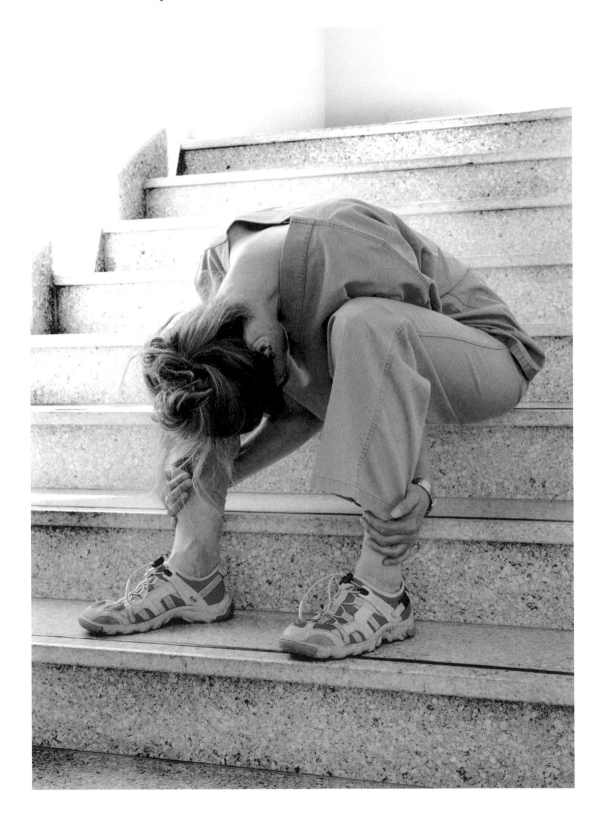

Inversions

The best known inversion is the head stand. For many laypersons, mastering the head, hand, or forearm stand equals mastering the entire yoga practice. The mountain posture, which was described in Chapter 7, leads to the ability to do a head stand. To achieve proper alignment this posture is combined with the child and tiger posture, as the flow from one posture into the other makes it easier to attain your goal. The turtle done in a seated posture on the chair (see "Yoga Exercises at Work") is also an inverted posture.

Their Purposes

In all inverted postures, the head is below heart level. The flow of the blood toward the heart is increased. If you stand on your legs for hours, you profit from the inverted posture—regardless of whether you lean your legs against a wall or do the head stand. The feeling of being able to turn things around can be experienced in all these postures. The shoulder stand is well known from sports classes.

Contraindications

People with uncontrolled high blood pressure or eye and ear conditions should not bow their heads below heart level.

Alignment

Make sure you put a bolster under your shoulders and save your neck from a harsh bend. The spinal column is stretched out as you know it from the upright stance. The pelvis is in an upright position and its muscles are tight. The knees are stretched without overdoing the stretch.

Half Shoulder Stand

- Lie on your back, bend both your knees, and place both your feet hip joint width apart on the ground. Your arms are stretched out at the sides of your body. Both palms are facing downward (Figure 8.16).
- Exhale and bring your knees to your chest and stretch your legs.

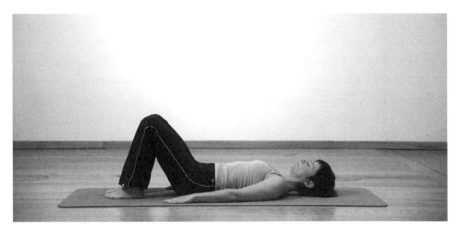

Figure 8.16. Half Shoulderstand

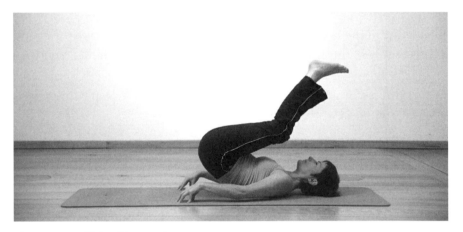

Figure 8.17. Half Shoulderstand

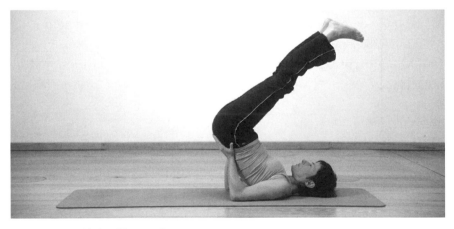

Figure 8.18. Half Shoulderstand

- Inhale and roll your spine upward, lifting your hips and lower torso. To support the lifting movement push your hands into the ground (Figure 8.17).
- To get into the posture place your hands at the top of your hips. Make sure your upper arms and elbows are parallel to the ground. Your feet are bent and the soles are pointing toward the ceiling (Figure 8.18).
- Maintain the position for six complete inhalations and exhalations.
- To get out of the posture, exhale while placing your hands at the sides of your body and lowering your spine vertebrae by vertebrae. Place your feet on the ground.
- Finally, stretch your legs and come into the starting position and feel the effects of the inversion. You may close your eyes if you like.
- As a counterstretch, assume the fish posture (see Figures 7.43 and 7.44).

Full Shoulder Stand

- Place a folded blanket on your mat and lie on your back. Your shoulders are at the edge of the folded blanket. Bend your knees and place both your feet hip joint width apart on the ground. Your arms are stretched out at the side of your body. Both palms are facing downward.
- Exhale and bring your knees to your chest and stretch your legs.
- Inhale and roll your spine upward, lifting your hips and torso. To support the lifting movement, push your hands into the ground. You can either do the complete stretch during one inhalation or raise your legs and torso in a couple of moves resting during exhalation.
- To get into the complete posture, place your hands at the top of your back. Make sure your upper arms and elbows are parallel to the ground. Your feet are bent and the soles are facing the ceiling (Figure 8.19).
- Maintain the position for six complete inhalations and exhalations.
- To get out of the posture exhale while placing your hands at the sides of your body and lowering your spine vertebrae by vertebrae. Place your feet on the ground.
- Finally, stretch your legs and come into the supine posture and feel the effects of the inversion. You may close your eyes if you like.
- As a counterstretch, assume the fish posture (see Figures 7.43 and 7.44).

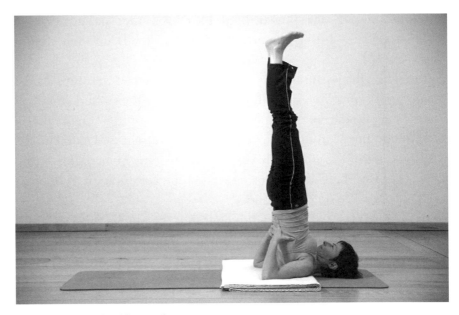

Figure 8.19. Full Shoulderstand

Twisted Postures

Rotations can be done in motion or as an asana. Rotations support the upright position and increase your flexibility. If you stretch out your vertebrae and concentrate on the movement, you become better aware of your polarity and your position in a given space. Rotations can counteract polarities and provide a feeling of relaxation and balance. They are ideal postures in an antistress program.

Their Purposes

Depending on the part of the spine that is being rotated, the stretch can be smaller or larger. Independently of the degree of the rotation, all vertebrae, muscles, discs, and tendons are addressed. Rotations straighten the spine and help prevent crooked postures (scoliosis).

You easily become aware of the missing flexibility of your upper torso while driving a car and looking over your shoulder. The torso rotation while opening to the side is a very good exercise with which to gain flexibility in the upper spine. The twisted triangle is a rotation of the lower spine and enhances the feeling of balance.

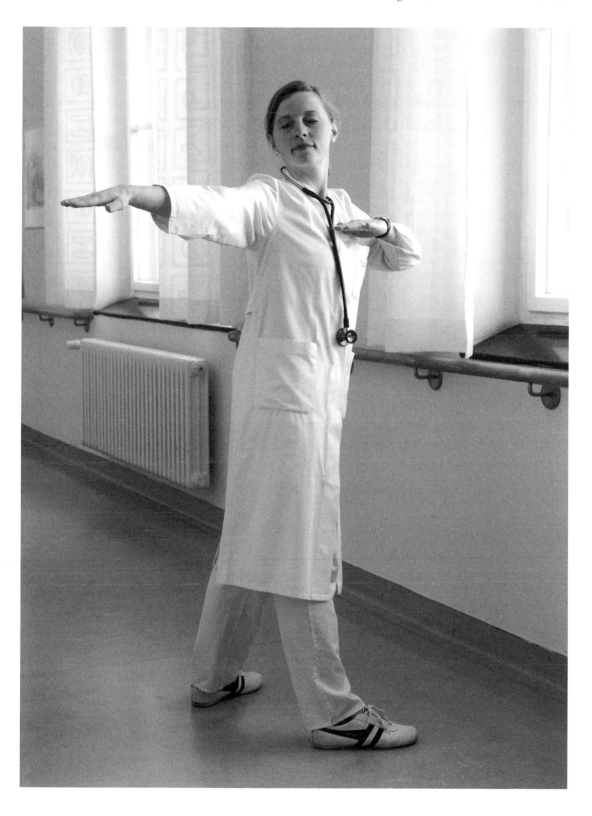

Contraindications

Avoid these exercises if you suffer from acute pain in your stomach or back. The detailed asana in this book are not designed for pregnant women. Twists as well as detox breathing (see Figures 7.28–7.32) are especially not advised for pregnant women.

Alignment

To be able to rotate the spine, it is necessary to stretch the complete spinal column and create space for the vertebrae and discs. All rotations should start with an inhalation and profound stretch.

Torso Rotation

- Come into the tiger posture (see the tiger posture). Place your forearms on your mat. Make sure that your elbows are underneath your shoulders and that your knees are underneath your hip joints. These alignments help you to exercise without hurting your joints (Figure 8.20).
- Inhale while you are rotating your upper torso and moving your left elbow upward (Figure 8.21).
- Exhale while moving back into the starting position.

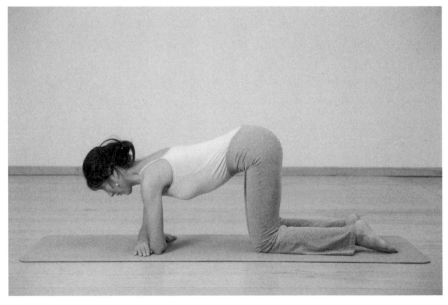

Figure 8.20. Torso Rotation

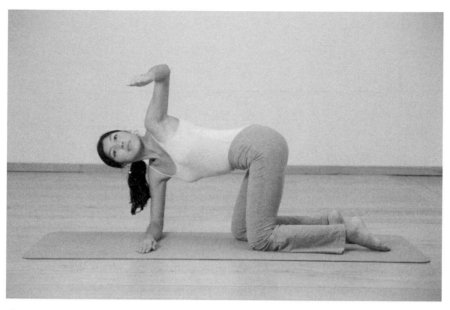

Figure 8.21. Torso Rotation

- Do the movement on both sides during six complete exhalations and inhalations.
- Finally, get back into the kneeling posture and place your hands on top of your thighs. Feel the effects with your eyes closed if you like.
- As a counterstretch, come into the child posture or the folded leaf posture (see Figure 7.45).

Twisted Triangle Posture

- Come into the standing posture. Place your feet one length of a leg apart. Turn your right foot outward with the toes pointing forward. Turn your left foot 45 degrees inward. Step a little backward with your right foot. (The right foot is on the same level as the heel of your left foot.)
- Inhale while slowly raising your arms over the sides until they are fully stretched out at shoulder height. Make sure that you do not pull up your shoulders. If you are not exactly sure, raise your shoulders briefly and let them sink again (Figure 8.22).
- Exhale and turn to the right and rotate your upper torso 180 degrees. Keep your arms stretched out at shoulder level.
- Inhale and stretch your spine in this position (Figure 8.23).

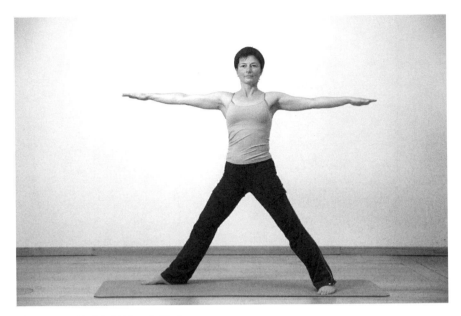

Figure 8.22. Twisted Triangle Posture

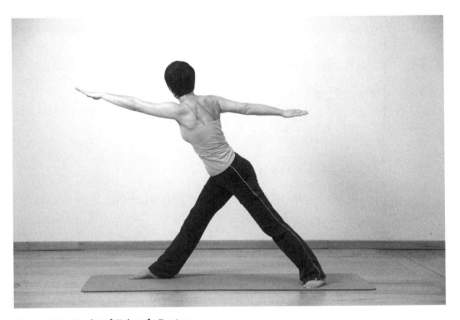

Figure 8.23. Twisted Triangle Posture

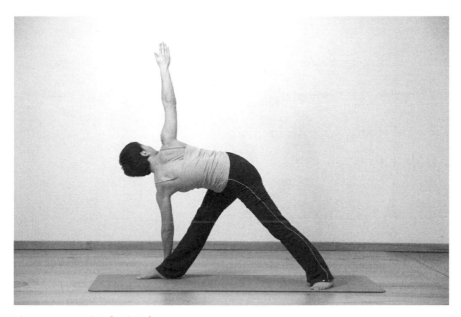

Figure 8.24. *Twisted Triangle Posture*

- Exhale and bend your torso to the side. Your left arm should move downward until your fingertips can reach the floor behind your front foot. Your right arm is stretched upward toward the ceiling. Make sure both arms are in line. Turn your head upward and look toward your upper hand (Figure 8.24).
- Maintain the twisted triangle posture for six complete inhalations and exhalations.
- To get out of the posture, inhale and rotate and lift your torso into the starting position.
- Lower your arms and hands with an exhalation.
- Close your eyes if you like and compare the feeling in both sides of your body: both legs, both sides of your pelvis, your shoulders, and both sides of your face.
- Repeat the posture on the other side.
- Finally, bring your feet closer together and feel the effects of the exercise in the standing posture. Close your eyes if it is pleasant for you.
- As a counterstretch, bend your knees. Exhale while bending your stretched torso forward. Relax your neck. Place your elbows on your knees or cross your arms and let them hang down.

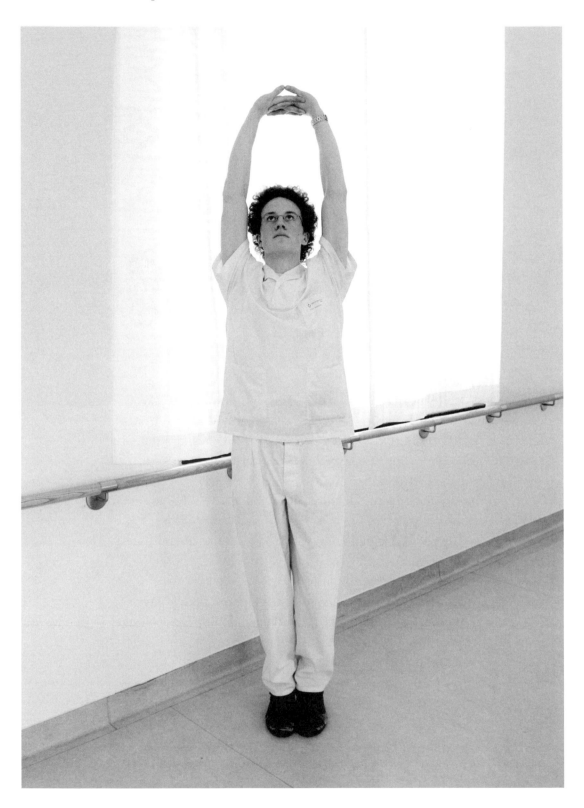

Balancing Postures

Two impressive balancing postures are the tree, with the person standing on one leg, and the eagle with the person standing on one foot with crossed legs and arms. Nevertheless, a balancing pose can also be a posture simply held on the tips of both feet, such as the palm tree posture, on one foot and one knee, such as the runner posture, or on both feet standing in line as in the forward bend posture (all these postures are detailed in Chapter 6, "Yoga Exercises at Work"). All balancing postures stretch the whole body, strengthen the feet and leg muscles, and help you to focus your attention.

Their Purposes

Balancing postures help to find the right combination of tension and relaxation. They tell you about your ability to maintain balance, be focused, and have a standing. The tree posture on one leg and the palm posture on the tips of your toes provide ideas for the successful management of stress: you can either resist stressful situations feeling like a rooted tree or you can elude stressful situations and feel like a swaying tree. The following two asana—the hero 3 posture and the eagle posture—describe the same effects.

Contraindications

There are no contraindications for the balancing postures, although they can be difficult to do. People who feel insecure while exercising in balancing postures should take hold of the back of a chair or lightly place a hand on a wall. You may need a lot of exercise to gain strength in your feet and legs and a lot of patience to stay in balance.

Alignment

To shift the balance to one foot or from the complete sole to the top of the toes requires a conscious movement supported by a profound breathing technique. Moving and breathing should be synchronized. To maintain good standing and to remain focused, it might be helpful to focus on an object at a distance.

Hero 3 Posture

- Come into the standing posture. Inhale while lifting your arms. Make sure your shoulders are relaxed (Figure 8.25).
- Shift your weight to your right leg and foot.
- Exhale while bending forward (Figure 8.26).
- In the alignment for the completed asana your arms, torso, and left leg are in line and parallel to the floor (Figure 8.27). You can either come into the posture during one exhalation or do a couple of moves, resting during inhalation.
- Maintain the posture for six complete inhalations and exhalations.
- Return to the starting position with an inhalation. Exhale and lower your arms over your sides.
- Close your eyes and compare the feeling in both sides of your body: both legs, both sides of your pelvis, your shoulders, and both sides of your face.
- Repeat the posture on the other side.
- Finally, feel the effects of the exercise in the standing posture. Close your eyes if it is pleasant for you.

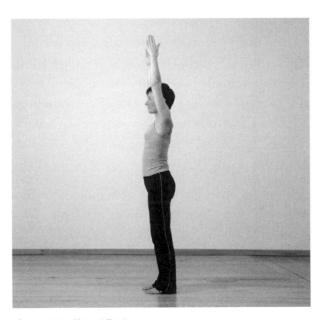

Figure 8.25. Hero 3 Posture

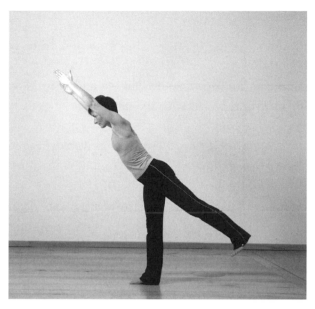

Figure 8.26. Hero 3 Posture

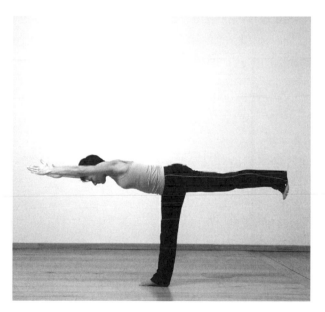

Figure 8.27. Hero 3 Posture

Variation: If you have trouble maintaining the posture—it could be a question of the strength of your feet and legs or your stability—exercise with the help of a chair. Place your fingertips on the back of a chair in front of you.

Eagle Posture

- Come into the standing posture. Shift your weight to your left foot and bend both knees.
- Inhale while you are lifting your right leg and cross it over your left leg. Keep your right leg next to the outer side of your left calf. Exhale and stabilize your position.
- Inhale while you are crossing your left forearm over your right forearm and bring your palms together in front of your stomach. Exhale and stabilize your position (Figure 8.28).
- Inhale while you are rotating your forearms inward until you can place your hands in front of your chest. Make sure that your palms are close together during the complete movement. Exhale and stabilize your position again (Figure 8.29).
- Inhale while you are rotating your forearms outward and stretch your arms until they are fully stretched out over your head. Make sure your palms are close together during the movement and that you do not pull up your shoulders. Exhale and stabilize your position (Figure 8.30).
- Maintain this posture for six complete inhalations and exhalations. Some people can stabilize their posture if they focus on a distant point.

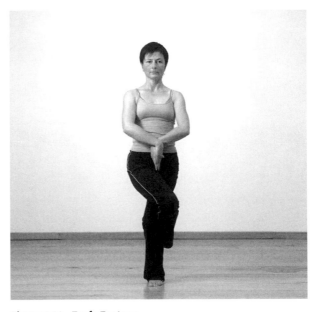

Figure 8.28. Eagle Posture

- Exhale while your are lowering your arms and right leg until you are again in the starting posture. Compare both sides: your legs, your shoulders and arms, and both sides of your face.
- Repeat the posture on the other side.

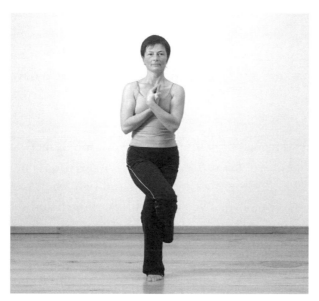

Figure 8.29. Eagle Posture

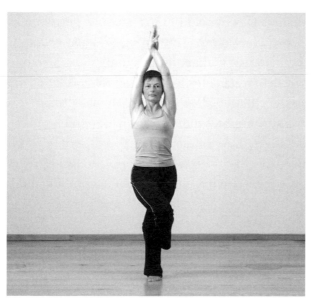

Figure 8.30. Eagle Posture

● Finally, come back into the starting position, compare both sides again, and feel the effects of the whole asana. Close your eyes if it is pleasant for you.

Eye Exercises

Eye exercises are special asana that train the muscles of your eyes. The eye exercises are also synchronized with your breathing. They can be done anywhere and should be done at least once a day.

Their Purposes

After staring at a computer screen all day, your eyes become tired and your vision can be temporarily blurry. If you have to focus your vision over a long period while working in artificial light, your eyes may burn and itch. The reason is that you do not blink enough and your eyes lose moisture. Unfortunately, a lot of our leisure time is spent in front of the television or the computer.

If your eyes are constantly at the same focus, your eye muscles are weakening in the same way that a constant seated position weakens your leg and stomach muscles. Most people do not realize that eye muscles also need a work out to stay flexible and maintain strength.

Yoga exercises help you to moisten your eyes, to switch from close viewing to distant viewing, and to extend your peripheral view. Regular exercises can also compensate for age-related vision loss and help you to maintain your visual acuity. You only need a couple of minutes to enable your ocular muscles to better adapt and help your eyes to remain moisturized. Better blood circulation and profound relaxation of the whole area surrounding your eyes provide good relief. Your eyes feel relaxed and energized. At the same time you experience a powerful anti-wrinkle effect. Together with adequate posture and proper breathing, eye exercises can also help you to better concentrate and focus again.

Contraindication

If you normally wear glasses, take them off while you are exercising. If you have serious eye problems such as glaucoma or macular degenerations you should talk to your doctor about the following exercises. For eye exercises, see Figures 6.12 to 6.18.

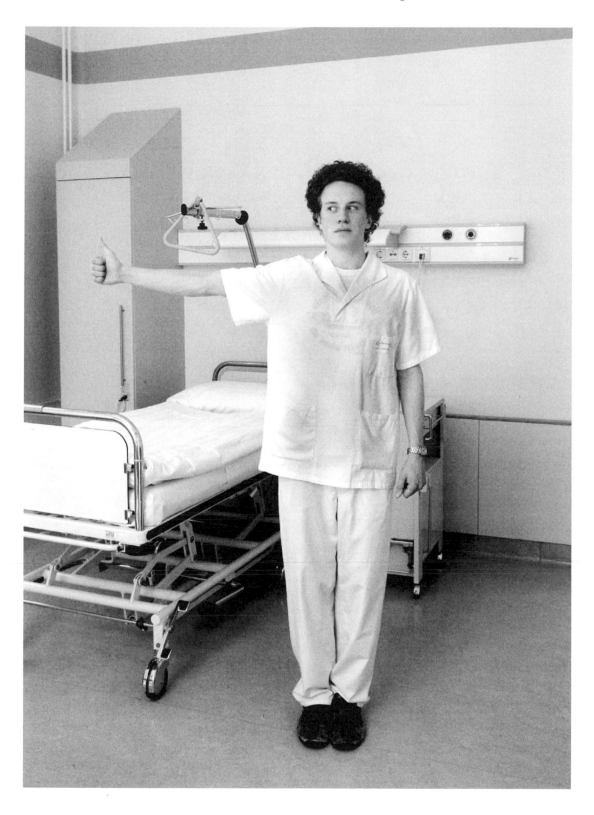

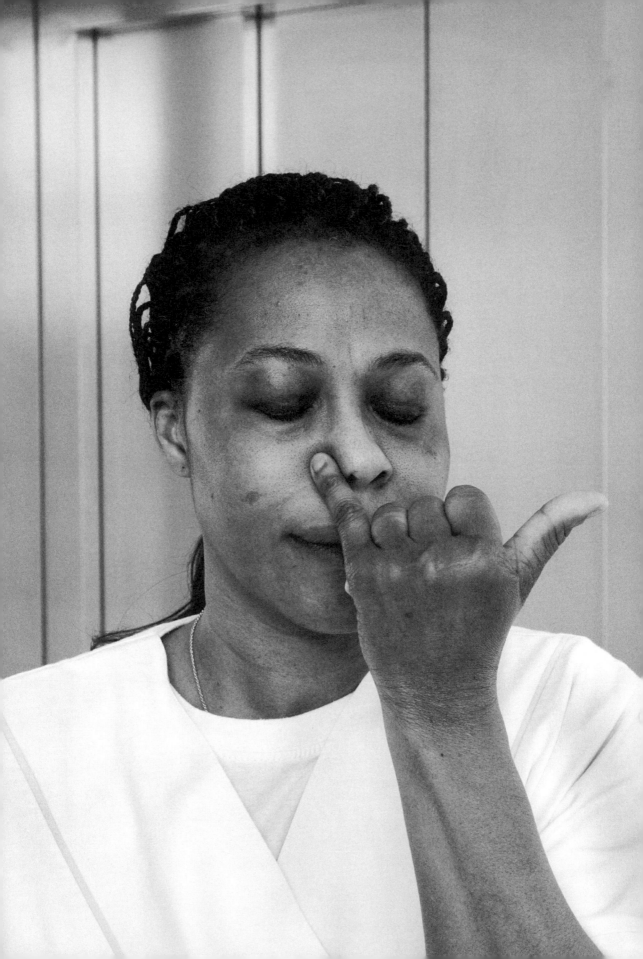

Concentration and Meditation

9

As a beginner, you will feel the effects of yoga while you are practicing some of the asana. They require all of your strength and attention. As a result, you build muscles and shape your body. At the same time, you relax and experience the freedom of your thinking. While practicing your asana, you are concentrating on your alignment and breath. This helps you to relax by shifting the focus of your thinking from your daily chores. At the end of a session, your mind is calm and you might find that your worries were set at rest. As a more advanced practitioner, it is easier to get into the asana and you acquire resources for a more profound practice. This is the right time to develop or deepen your practice of pranayama and meditation.

To introduce meditating as a state of consciousness, it might be helpful for you to place it into the context of being asleep and being awake. (Transcendental meditation differentiates four states of mind: being awake, dreaming, sleeping, and meditating.) The question is: In which ways is meditating different from being awake or being asleep?

If you think of being open minded, being conscious, and being relaxed as three mental qualities, you obtain different results regarding the three states of mind. The following might provide a first overview of the interrelations.

The Effects of Meditation

Western medicine and alternative therapy both recommend meditation as a relaxing technique. Brain waves are altered while people are meditating, their heart beats are slower, their breathing is deeper, and their muscles are more relaxed.

Meta-analysis of studies on meditation and physical or psychic phenomenon state the evidence for the positive effects of meditation, but also mention the lack of scientific standards. The influence of meditation varies as do the conditions of the people practicing meditation. This makes it difficult to find causal connections.

Nevertheless, there is no doubt about either the positive effects of meditation on the body and mind or the fact that meditation requires a lot of practicing before you can benefit from it. If you have already experienced meditative moments practicing asana and pranayama, you are well prepared for the next step.

State of Consciousness	Mental Quality		
	Being Open Minded	*Being Conscious*	*Being Relaxed*
Sleeping	Yes *Anything might happen in our dreams.*	No *Sleeping is the opposite of being conscious.*	Yes and No *A good sleep is relaxing, but sleep can also be stressful and intimidating: people chew on their teeth while sleeping or suddenly wake up from fearful dreams.*
Being Awake	Yes and No *Depending on the issue, the way we are approached, and the individual resources.*	Yes *We ignore the moments of absent mindedness and think of them as exceptions.*	Yes and No *This book is meant to help you in being relaxed in stressful situations. Unfortunately, as long as we live we always experience situations and moments that are stressful and that we can hardly cope with.*
Meditating	Yes *Being able to meditate involves opening up to thoughts and feelings.*	Yes *Most obviously in active forms of meditation: asana, pranayama, and reciting or singing mantras.* *But also while meditating and listening to sounds and focusing on objects, inner pictures, or your own breathing.*	Yes *Meditation leads to a profound state of tranquility and relaxation.*

Some Techniques of Meditation

It is a popular misconception that meditating is something passive. People think of the diverse statues of Buddha sitting in the lotus posture. This is a well-known posture and one way in which you can meditate. But you can differentiate active and passive forms of meditation. The most obvious active forms of meditation are reciting, singing, and walking—or doing asana and pranayama.

The already mentioned Yoga-Sutras speak of the eights limbs of yoga:

Yama	Ethical behavior (i.e., nonviolence, truthfulness)
Niyama	Personal behavior (i.e., cleanliness, spiritual austerities)
Asana	Postures
Pranayama	Breathing exercises
Pratyahara	Withdrawal of the senses from the external world, sensory inhibition
Dharana	Withdrawal from the distractions of the mind, concentration
Dhyana	Continuous flow of concentration, meditation
Samadi	Highest form of being, thinking, and feeling, ecstasy

As you can see, there is not just one way of concentrating and meditating, just as there is no steady way forward from one to eight. Rather, there are diverse states of mind and being. Since our aim is to learn to focus and relax, we will concentrate on Pratyahara, Dharana, and techniques of withdrawing from the outside world. In this way, we will learn to concentrate on ourselves or to think about nothing at all.

Walking Meditation

Walking can be a good way to withdraw your attention from outside stimuli and direct your attentions to your inner self. While you are aware and feel the way you walk—the pressure on your soles, the warmth of your feet, the movement of your knees, and so on—you detach yourself from the outside. This experience of self-concentration needs a protected space, such as a park, a path through an apartment, or just a circle in a room.

Walking and jogging have these calming and focusing elements. Unfortunately, these techniques, as well as many other fitness exercises, often lack body awareness as a first step to concentrating and meditating. People exercise without noticing what they are doing; they listen to music while ruining their hips and knees because of incorrect walking, wearing the wrong shoes, and so on.

The easiest way to find out if walking is an appropriate way to meditate is to practice and experience it. If you think about walking in a positive manner, you should try it out and walk a little path for 20 to 30 minutes. Keep your attention focused on all aspects of the walking activity. Note how long you can keep your attention focused and honor your new ability.

Meditation on Your Body

We take it for granted that we function every day. We complain about pain or being unable to stretch or relax and often do not notice how we have harmed ourselves. Give your body profound thought and praise it. Your thoughts can either "walk" through your body from tip to toe and praise it, that is, your feet that carry you along every day, your stomach that digests healthy and unhealthy food, your ears that help you listen and connect to others, and so on. Or you can concentrate on one organ, one part of your body, and think about it, feel it, and honor it.

A well known technique in yoga is the yoga nidra. To learn it, you lie down in shanti asana and become aware of your body part by part. You start out with your little toe of your left foot, the toe next to it, the middle toe, the toe next to it, the big toe, the sole, the heel, etc. until you come to your face, your left eyebrow, your left eye, and so on. Since there is generally no correct way of doing this, just a personal way for each of us, you should just try it out. You will find that this technique is also very helpful if you have problems sleeping. Of cause you can buy a recording and get an introduction or learn in a yoga group. Listening to someone "walking" through a body is different and also very relaxing.

Mantra Meditation

A mantra can be a syllable, a word, a line, a poem, or a song. The most famous mantra in yoga is "OM." There are diverse interpretations of "OM" depending on the belief of the writer. Undoubtedly, OM sounds wonderful and could be considered "the sound of all sounds." OM can be recited or sung (either in your mind or aloud), alone and in groups, with all singing at a time or as a canon. Another very well-known mantra of Hinduism is the Gayatri Mantra, a hymn to the God of the light. You can receive the text, the proper pronunciation, and the rhythm if you type "gayatri" into a search engine.

The sound of "hamsa" is connected to breathing. In yoga, hamsa is called "the unpronounced mantra" because it "is continually produced by the body as a result of the breathing process. The syllable ham is connected with inhalation, sa with exhalation" (Feuerstein, 2000). All you have to do is to think or say ham while you are inhaling and sa while you are exhaling.

But you can also choose one word with an important connotation for you. It could be a word in English, such as silence, love, or confidence, or a word in Sanskrit, such as *citi-shakti* (power of awareness) or ananda (bliss); you can then recite this word again and again. You can do the same with a line of a poem or a complete poem. It just needs your resolution and your patience to try it out. Keep to your mantra and repeat it again and again for a certain time. If negative thoughts arise, repeat your mantra. In case you do not recognize a negative thought, ask yourself if a particular thought is helpful. If your thought is not helpful, get rid of it with the help of your mantra.

Sound Meditation

Yoga is closely connected with the sound of singing bowls. These bowls can be made of metal or glass. Depending on the material of the bowl and the drumstick you get different sounds: a short ringing or a long lasting sound. This kind of listening to a sound can be done in groups or practiced alone. You concentrate on the sound as long as possible. Become aware of the time you can focus your mind on listening to the sound and refocus when you are withdrawing from it.

Visual Meditation

A yogi (more often you see a yogini—a woman practicing yoga) sitting in front of a candle meditating is also a common picture of yoga. Instead of a candle, you can take any object or a photo, a color, a written word on paper, or just a relaxing picture you have in your mind. Focus your attention on the object. See it in reality or in your mind and keep to it. Concentrate on the vision as long as possible. Become aware of the time you can focus your attention on this object or on your inner picture.

Thinking Nothing at All

You might feel that you cannot recall an address or a word and that your head is just empty. These thoughts and feelings do not result from a lack of information but from an overflow of information, data, appointments, contacts, and talks to which we are exposed. It is difficult to discriminate important and unimportant information. We are used to thinking about a few things at a time. While we are thinking "I must not forget to . . . " we are talking to someone, working, driving, and so on. To be able to do things unconsciously is helpful—otherwise we could not breathe and walk and think and talk all at the same time.

The art of Dharana involves the ability to give your thoughts a break, to stop listening, stop talking, and stop thinking. Learn to experience a profound pause—leave it all behind. To experience this you need to practice some of the other meditation techniques. Thinking nothing at all can follow one of the abovementioned meditative techniques or can be done just by itself: sitting and thinking nothing.

Your Meditative Practice

The following overview gives you a preliminary idea about how you could develop your own relaxing and meditative practice that could become part of your yoga program. You combine relaxing and balancing asana and pranayama exercises with one of the techniques described.

Introduction	Seated Posture
Balancing Asana	Shoulder Bridge
	Crocodile Posture
Pranayama	Alternate Nostril Breathing
Meditation on Your body	
Mantra Meditation	Seated Posture: Free Seat or Lotus Seat
Sound Meditation	Supine Posture: Shanti Asana
Visual Meditation	
Thinking Nothing at All	
Conclusion	Seated Posture

All postures have already been introduced in Chapter 7, "Yoga Exercises at Home," except for the alternate nostril breathing, which was described in Chapter 6, "Yoga Exercises at Work." If you become aware of a favorite meditation technique, you can look for more specific literature concerning it.

Enjoy yourself meditating. Learn to be patient with yourself and honor each step of your progress.

Addresses and Literature 10

Yoga Traditions and Their Websites

Note: All Websites were last accessed on October 9, 2008.

Anusara: www.anusara.com
Ashtanga: www.ashtanga.com
Bikram: www.bikramyoga.com
Gitananda: www.gitanandayogasociety.com
Iyengar: www.iynaus.org
Jivamukti: www.jivamuktiyoga.com
Kundalini: www.3ho.org
Sivananda: www.sivananda.org
Triyoga: www.triyoga.com
Vini: www.viniyoga.com

Literature

Austin, M. (2004). *Cool Yoga Tricks.* (New York: Ballantine Books).

Carrico, M. (1997). *Yoga Journal's Yoga Basics: The Essential Beginner's Guide to Yoga for a Lifetime of Health and Fitness.* (New York: Owl Book).

Coulter, H. D. (2001). *Anatomy of Hatha Yoga. A Manual for Students, Teachers, and Practitioners.* (Honesdale, PA: Body and Breath).

Ebert, D. (2003). Westliche Medizin und Yoga. In: *Der Weg des Yoga. Handbuch für Übende und Lehrende.* (Petersberg: Via Nova), pp. 275–285.

Feuerstein, G. (2000). *The Shambhala Encyclopedia of Yoga.* (Boston, London: Shambhala).

Snyder, M., and Lindquist, R. (2006). *Complementary/Alternative Therapies in Nursing.* (New York: Springer Publishing Company).

Index

Acute pain, 31, 174

Advanced practitioner, 148,188

Alignment, 10, 30, 53, 59, 85, 91, 95, 110, 114, 124–128, 130, 148, 151, 157, 161, 164, 169, 174, 179, 188

Alternate nostril breathing posture, 31–32, 75–77, 82, 194

Arm rotation posture, 32, 47–48

Asana, 8, 14, 18, 30, 32, 69, 80, 148. *See* Postures

Awareness, 9, 10, 31, 80, 82–83, 88, 90–91, 110. *See* Consciousness

Back
  aches, 80, 86, 151
  lower, 32, 53–59, 82, 94
  upper, 32, 46–51, 157, 161

Backward bends, 155–160

Balance, 5, 10, 30, 65–69, 73, 82, 172, 179

Balancing postures, 178–184

Basic stances, 31–32, 84–90

Beginner of yoga, 30, 81, 188

Bend and twist, 32, 69–71

Blood pressure, high, 30, 54, 85–86, 91, 94–95, 123, 127, 151, 169

Boat posture, 83, 136–137

Bow posture
  lying, 148, 155, 159–160
  standing, 148, 157–159

Breathing, 4, 8–10, 14, 18–19, 31, 80 84, 90–91, 179, 184. *See* Pranayama

Camel posture, 82, 109, 116–117

Child posture, 83, 123–128, 130

Clothes for yoga practice, 24, 80

Cobra posture, 82, 105–106

Concentration, 8, 20, 32, 73–77, 186–194. *See* Meditation

Consideration, 30–31, 80

Consciousness, 14, 21, 30, 148, 188–189

Contraindications, 84–85, 91, 94, 110, 123

Counteract, 8, 9, 20, 31

Counterstretch, 107, 153, 155, 159, 161, 165, 167, 171, 175, 177

Cow posture, 83, 138–139

Crocodile posture, 83, 142–144, 194
  easy crocodile posture, 82, 94, 96

Cupping and blinking posture, 32, 44–46, 149

Detox breathing posture, 82, 111–114

Dorsal arm and leg stretch posture, 82, 94, 98–99

Eagle posture, 149, 179, 182–184

Ear conditions, 151, 169

Eight limbs of yoga, 190

Elephant posture, 31, 35–37

Energy, 8, 30, 32, 65–69, 73, 149, 155

Exercises, 19–21, 148, 161. *See* Postures

Eyes
  burning, 41–46
  conditions, 151, 169
  moisturized, 41–46
  peripheral view, 41–43
  yoga exercises, 32, 41–46, 149, 184–185

Feeling blue, 33, 69–73

Feet, tired, 32, 60, 63–65

Fingers, stiff, 47, 51–53

Fish posture, 83, 109, 121–122

Folded leaf posture, 83, 112, 128, 130, 194

Forward bending, 32, 55–57

Forward bends, 149–155

Free seat posture, 82–83, 88, 145

Goals, personal, 25–26

Great gesture posture, 32, 48–49, 82, 118–119

Half lotus posture, 82–84, 89, 144

Half moon posture, 148, 163–165

Hand gesture posture, 32, 51–52

Hand lotus posture, 32, 52–53

Hands, hurting, 46, 51–53
Hatha Yoga, 14–18
Hatha Yoga Pradipika, 15
Headaches, 8, 31, 36
Head bow posture, 31, 37–39
Head rotation posture, 31, 37–38
Head to knee posture, 148, 151–153
Hernia, 31
Hero 1 posture, 32, 65–68
Hero 2 posture, 32, 71–72
Hero 3 posture, 149, 179–181
Hip
    joints, 82, 94–95
    rotation posture, 81–82, 95, 99–102

Inflammation, 31
Inversions, 168–172

Journal, personal, 25–27

Kneeling posture, 82–83, 86–87, 145
Knee rotation posture, 32, 60–61
Knee to chest posture, 82, 94, 96–97
Knees
    stiff, 32, 59–61
    pain, 82

Leg lift sideways posture, 82, 95, 102–103
Legs, tired, 32, 59–60, 62–63
Lotus seat posture, 82, 89–90, 145, 194
Lying eight posture, 32, 41–43, 149
Lying on the back posture, 82, 85–86

Meditation, 188–194
Memory, improve, 32, 73–77
Moody, 32, 69–73
Mountain posture, 83, 123–124, 126–127, 130
easy mountain posture, 32, 53–55
Muscles
    activity, 8
    pain, 5
    tension, 8, 18
    underdeveloped, 149, 155

Near and distant view posture, 32, 41, 43–44, 149
Neck, stiff, 31, 36–41, 157, 161

Palm posture
    on the floor, 82
    standing, 32, 59, 63–65
Patanjali, 15
Pelvis, 82, 94, 149

Posture, poor, 32, 46, 53, 65, 149, 157, 161
Postures
    alternate nostril breathing, 31–32, 75–77, 82, 194
    arm rotation, 32, 47–48
    basic stances, 31–32, 84–90
    bend and twist, 32, 69–71
    boat, 83, 136–137
    bow
        lying, 148, 155, 159–160
        standing, 148, 157–159
    camel, 82, 109, 116–117
    child, 83, 123–128, 130
    cobra, 82, 105–106
    cow, 83, 138–139
    crocodile, 83, 142–144, 194
        easy crocodile, 82, 94, 96
    cupping and blinking, 32, 44–46, 149
    detox breathing, 82, 111–114
    dorsal arm and leg stretch, 82, 94, 98–99
    eagle, 149, 179, 182–184
    elephant, 31, 35–37
    fish, 83, 109, 121–122
    folded leaf, 83, 112, 128, 130, 194
    forward bending, 32, 55–57
    free seat, 82–83, 88, 145
    great gesture, 32, 48–49, 82, 118–119
    half lotus, 82–84, 89, 144
    half moon, 148, 163–165
    half shoulder stand, 148
    hand gesture, 32, 51–52
    hand lotus, 32, 52–53
    head bow, 31, 37–39
    head rotation, 31, 37–38
    head to knee, 148, 151–153
    hero 1, 32, 65–68
    hero 2, 32, 71–72
    hero 3, 149, 179–181
    hip rotation, 81–82, 95, 99–102
    kneeling, 82–83, 86–87, 145
    knee rotation, 32, 60–61
    knee to chest, 82, 94, 96–97
    leg lift sideways, 82, 95, 102–103
    lotus seat, 82, 89–90, 145, 194
    lying eight, 32, 41–43, 149
    lying on the back, 82, 85–86
    mountain, 83, 123–124, 126–127, 130
        easy mountain, 32, 53–55
    near and distant view, 32, 41, 43–44, 149
    palm
        on the floor, 82
        standing, 32, 59, 63–65
    pyramid, 83, 123, 132–133

runner, 32, 59, 62–63, 83, 123, 130–131

seated, 31, 34–35, 82, 87, 194

shanti asana, 82, 83, 90–92, 144, 194

shoulder bridge, 83, 140–141, 194

shoulder stand
  full, 148, 171–172
  half, 148, 169–171

side angle, 148, 165–167

sphinx, 82, 105–107

spider, 82, 107–109

standing, 31, 33–34

stargazer, 32, 68–69

sunbird, 83, 123–124, 127

table, 83,120–121

threading the needle, 83, 128–129

tiger, 83, 123, 125–128

tiger breathing, 82, 114–115

torso rotation, 172, 174–175
  standing, 32, 49–50, 149

tree, 32, 72–75
  on the floor, 82, 91–94

triangle, 83, 134–136
  in motion, 32, 57–59
  twisted, 149, 172, 175–177

turtle, 148, 153–155
  easy turtle, 31, 40, 168–189

ventral arms and legs stretch, 81–82, 95, 104–105

Practice, individual, 19–21, 30, 81

Pranayama, 82–83, 109–110, 188, 194. *See* Breathing

Pregnant women and yoga, 30, 174

Props for yoga, 25, 80, 86

Pyramid posture, 83, 123, 132–133

Runner posture, 32, 59, 62–63, 83, 123, 130–131

Sanskrit, 14–15

Sciatica, 31

Seated posture, 31, 34–35, 82, 87, 194

Self
  attention, 10
  efficacy, 10–11

Schools, 14–15, 18, 20, 24, 123. *See* Traditions of yoga; Style

Shanti asana posture, 82, 83, 90–92, 144, 194

Shoulder bridge posture, 83, 140–141, 194

Shoulders
  mobility, 94
  stiff, 31–32, 36–41, 82
  poor posture, of 46–51

Shoulder stand posture
  full, 148, 171–172
  half, 148, 169–171

Side angle posture, 148, 165–167

Sideward bends, 161–167

Sphinx posture, 82, 105–107

Spider posture, 82, 107–109

Standing posture, 31, 33–34

Stargazer posture, 32, 68–69

Stress, 8–10, 27, 31, 172, 179

Style, 14–15, 18, 20, 123. *See* Traditions of yoga; Schools

Sunbird posture, 83, 123–124, 127

Surgery, yoga after, 31

Table posture, 83,120–121

Teachers of yoga, 18, 24

Tension, 8–10
  relief, 35, 82, 110–111, 179

Threading the needle posture, 83, 128–129

Tiger posture, 83, 123, 125–128

Tiger breathing posture, 82, 114–115

Time to practice, 18, 20, 80–81, 94, 144

Torso rotation posture, 149, 172, 174–175
  standing, 32, 49–50

Tree posture, 32, 72–75
  on the floor, 82, 91–94

Triangle posture, 83, 134–136
  in motion, 32, 57–59
  twisted, 149, 172, 175–177

Traditions of yoga, 14–15, 18, 20, 196. *See* Schools; Style

Turtle posture, 148, 153–155
  easy turtle posture, 31, 40, 168–189

Twisted postures, 172–177

Ventral arms and legs stretch posture, 81–82, 95, 104–105

Wrists
  hurting, 32, 47

Yoga Sutras, 14–15, 190